RODALE'S
ESSENTIAL
HERBAL
HANDBOOKS

Herbal Home Hints

HUNDREDS OF TIPS AND FORMULAS FOR CLEANING JUST ABOUT ANYTHING

Louise Gruenberg

Rodale Press, Inc.
Emmaus, Pennsylvania

Dedicated to the health and happiness of all beings, and especially created for all the women in my life — past, present, and future.

OUR PURPOSE

"We inspire and enable people to improve their lives and the world around them."

Storey Books:
Editor: Gwen W. Steege
Text Designer: Eugenie Seidenberg Delaney
Cover Designer: Meredith Maker
Text Illustrators: All illustrations by Beverly K. Duncan with the exception of those by Sarah Brill, pages 5, 29, 30, 33, 40 (top and bottom), 51, 54, 56; Brigita Fuhrmann, pages 2, 36, 39, 48, 58; Charles Joslin, pages 28, 32 (bottom), 35, 41, 44, 45, 50, 55, 57; and Mallory Lake, pages 15, 37, 47, 49
Production Assistant: Susan Bernier
Indexer: Susan Olason, Indexes and Knowledge Maps

Rodale Press Garden Books:
Executive Editor: Ellen Phillips
Editor: Karen Costello Soltys
Executive Creative Director: Christin Gangi
Art Director and Cover Designer: Patricia Field
Cover Illustrator: Mia Bosna
Studio Manager: Leslie Keefe
Manufacturing Manager: Mark Krahforst

For questions or comments concerning the editorial content of this book, please write to:
Rodale Press, Inc.
Book Readers' Service
33 East Minor Street
Emmaus, PA 18098
For more information about Rodale Press and the books and magazines we publish, visit our World Wide Web site at:
http://www.rodalepress.com

Library of Congress Cataloging-in-Publication Data
Gruenberg, Louise M.
    Herbal home hints / Louise Gruenberg.
       p.   cm. — (Rodale's essential herbal handbooks)
    Includes index.
    ISBN 0-87596-814-7 (alk. paper)
    1. House cleaning. 2. Herbs. 3. Recipes. I. Title. II. Series.
    TX324 .G78 1999
    648'.5—dc21   99–6001

ISBN 0-87596-814-7 hardcover   ISBN 0-87596-830-9 paperback
Distributed in the book trade by St. Martin's Press
Printed in the United States
2 4 6 8 10 9 7 5 3 1 hardcover
2 4 6 8 10 9 7 5 3 1 paperback

Contents

CHAPTER 1

HERBAL
Housekeeping

Too busy to clean? These formulas can actually save you time, as well as money, while providing you with safe products that solve all kinds of household problems. Most of my cleaning formulas are simple to make and can be prepared in advance to be stored, conveniently ready for use as needed. With them, you can make your home a sweet-smelling haven for you and your family.

Cleaning with herbs is not only easy and effective, but it's also good for our earth. With the information and formulas in this book, you will soon be an expert at using herbs to clean just about anything, even if you've never used herbs in this way before.

An Invitation

Like me, you may find the repetitiveness of housecleaning boring. But I feel calmer when my house is clean, and I am better able to cope with the demands of my life when it is tidy, sensibly organized, and beautiful. To help make everyday chores more enjoyable, I've researched and experimented for more than 25 years, finding new ways to use the aromatic herbs and essential oils I love. Through this process, I've had the pleasure of making the mundane magical as I've learned to use some of nature's finest fragrances. My "cleaning team" is Rose, Melissa, Rosemary, Basil, and other herbs, whose scents sweeten my tasks and whose virtues protect my family. It's a tribute to the herbs and gratifying to me that, no matter the season, guests almost always tell us how wonderful our home smells.

What is less evident, but perhaps more important, is that the same herbs that provide sensory pleasure also combat all kinds of nasty microorganisms lurking about on the surfaces and in the air of our homes. Hyssop, mints, lavender, roses, lemon balm, sage, thyme — all of these herbs and many others have been used for centuries to clean and freshen. Unlike chemical cleansers, the aromatic herbs and natural minerals that are the best, most ecological cleaners don't have a press agency to tout their virtues, so I am speaking for them.

Hyssop

A GARDEN OF HOUSEKEEPING HERBS

The source for many of my housekeeping herbs is my herb garden, which surrounds our city home with fragrant greenery. Roses with a recurrent blooming habit climb the south walls, lavender edges some of the bark-chip paths, lady's mantle and lemon thyme edge others. The groundcovers in the front-yard perennial beds are lemon mint, orange mint, and peppermint. The backyard is a riot of elecampane, coneflowers, comfrey, and many other medicinal herbs.

I enrich my soil organically, and it rewards me with strong plants that require little care from me, and with abundant crops, which I use as flavorings, teas, medicines, craft materials, and in my household cleaning products. I feel a strong connection to the earth through this wise use of its renewable resources.

AN OVERVIEW OF THE BOOK

In the pages that follow, I'll share with you much of what I've learned about growing and using herbs. In Chapter 2, Supplies and Methods, you'll begin your herbal housekeeping education by learning about the supplies and equipment you'll need, along with simple, basic methods for formulating home care products.

Chapter 3, Housekeeping Herbs A to Z, is an alphabetical directory of 34 herbs, with descriptions of their antiseptic, antiviral, insect-repellent, or fixative possibilities, as well as advice on growing or buying them, and how to process them.

If you decide to grow your housekeeping herbs, Chapter 4, Growing Herbs for Cleaning, provides everything you need to get started with annual, tender perennial, and perennial herbs. You will also learn when to collect your herbs and how to prepare, dry, and store your herbs. Several herb garden designs, including container garden plans, will help you integrate a beautiful and useful garden into your own yard, porch, patio, or deck.

In Chapter 5, Herbal Housekeeping Recipes, you'll find dozens of formulas developed to clean and care for everything from glass and metal to carpets and leather. Many of the formulas suggest weekly variations that use different essential oils to increase the bacteria-fighting ability of the products and prevent the development of bacteria resistance. This chapter also contains some quick, easy, and fun projects for sachets, air fresheners, insect pest deterrents, and simmering potpourris. The chapter concludes with important reference charts describing herbal housekeeping ingredients, including essential oils and fixatives, their uses, and where to find them (pages 136–45).

HERBAL TRADITIONS

As John Parkinson wrote in 1629, "Many herbs and flowers with their fragrant smells do comfort, and as it were revive the spirits and perfume the whole house." Long before supermarkets and modern manufacturers of cleaning products existed, people got by with what they could grow, make, or trade. Nine out of ten of them were employed in agricultural pursuits and thus were likely to recognize an herb that grew in the meadow, hedgerow, or woods, and to know a good bit about its uses.

In the Middle Ages, when most cottages had floors of pounded earth, householders brought fresh plant material indoors to strew around, providing a pleasant softness underfoot and perfuming the dark and smoky interior. The plants served to keep insect populations somewhat under control, too. Wealthy people carried pomanders of ambergris, musk, orange, and spices, or wore them around their necks or waists to protect against disease. Herbs even found their way into courtrooms: Bouquets of rue, rosemary, southernwood, and other herbs were set about to protect the judge from the dreaded jail fever.

In today's world, whenever I'm faced with a pile of laundry, a dirty bathroom, a messy kitchen, and a job deadline of one sort or another, I remember those long-ago efforts, and I comfort myself with the thought that it could be much worse. The deadline still requires energy and discipline, but thanks to modern sanitation and

Soapy Waters

Commercial soap did not become widely available until the early 19th century. So what did people clean with before that? Plant ashes were used to make lye, urine was aged for its ammonia content, and, if they could afford it, women used vinegar. Small wonder that herbs were appreciated for their fragrance and use in "sweete washing waters"!

technology, there are so many things I don't have to do to get my house and clothes clean. Take, for example, clean hot water: How easy it is to take its availability for granted!

CREATING A NEW TRADITION

Like my ancestors, however, I like natural materials. And as you will see, many herbs have qualities that can help you clean, disinfect, scent your home, and deter pests. Plus, you can enhance the power of these herbs by blending materials like vinegar, alcohol, minerals, and essential oils with them.

Vinegar. One of the most natural partners for herbs is vinegar, because its acidity makes it a natural disinfectant: Bacteria prefer a more alkaline environment. Herbal vinegars have a long history. One early example is known as "The Four Thieves' Vinegar," which contained angelica, lavender, calamus, and rue. By drinking this concoction, and probably also carrying along a cloth saturated with it to smell, thieves could safely go among victims of the Great Plague of London in 1665 and loot without becoming infected. Now, that's potent stuff!

Lavender

Other solutions. You can also extract herbs in water, glycerin, or alcohols of various sorts: grain, isopropyl, or denatured grain. Occasionally, herbs are infused directly in oils. Adding 3 percent essential oil to a fixed oil is an easier, faster, but more expensive, way to achieve an effect similar to that of an infused oil without all the work. The solution you choose depends on the end use of the product.

Minerals. Herbs can also be combined with minerals, like baking soda, washing soda, salt, various clays, chalk, and others to do their work. I like to use them with natural soaps, including Murphy's Oil Soap, which is made from pine bark; Dr. Bronner's Liquid Castile Soaps; and, occasionally, grated bar soaps.

Essential oils: Essential oils concentrate the cleaning and disinfecting powers of plants. I blend purchased oils with liquid soaps, then add them to solutions they are soluble in: glycerin, alcohol, or oil. Of course, I also use them in potpourri and evaporate them in diffusers. Their intense fragrances can be overpowering, but when they are used properly they add a wonderful, welcoming ambiance. I consider the use of essential oils aromatherapy for my home, but everyone in the house benefits from their fragrant ability to raise the spirits while they disinfect.

For me, the fragrances of the herbs and essential oils, and the interesting blends I develop with them, make housekeeping less of a chore and more of a pleasurable, sensory experience. I hope you will find some formulas in this collection that make you feel the same way. You'll soon find that you're saving money by not buying cleaning products, even though you may be spending some of what you save on essential oils and herbs. As far as I'm concerned, it's a great trade-off!

Caution: Chemicals at Work

Today, the average home in the United States contains more chemicals than were found in a typical 19th-century chemistry lab. In fact, estimates project that every home uses 25 gallons of hazardous chemicals each year, and has from 50 to 100 pounds of dangerous materials requiring professional hazardous-waste disposal sitting around the kitchen, bathroom, basement, and garage. At the same time, 15 percent of the U.S. population is sensitive to chemicals in common household products, and evidence is mounting that this witches' brew of chemicals in our environment is responsible for chronic, long-term health effects of a serious nature for many more of us.

CHAPTER 2

SUPPLIES AND
Methods

T he basic methods I use are so simple that everyone can make their own cleaning products. It's easier than cooking, and there's less that can go wrong. Most of the time, you will be adding herbs — either fresh or dried, and sometimes a combination of the two — to a solvent, such as water, vinegar, alcohol, glycerin, ammonia, or oil. The basic formulas are on pages 19–26.

Most of the materials I use to make my herbal home products can be readily purchased at your local pharmacy, or grocery, hardware, paint, or health food store. For bulk purchases of herbs and other natural products, including essential oils, flower essences, and some fixed oils, check Herbal Resources, starting on page 146, for mail-order suppliers.

Basic Equipment for Herbal Formulas

You may already have everything you need in your kitchen to make herbal cleaning supplies. If not, you can probably improvise some items and purchase others. In this section, I'll tell you about the kitchenware needed to make any of the formulas in the book. Depending upon which types of formulas you intend to make and use, you may not need everything described here.

The equipment used to process herbal formulas should be made of glass, heat-treated glass, glass-ceramic fusions (such as Corningware), ceramic (nonleaded glazes), enameled steel, enameled cast iron, or stainless steel. These materials are less reactive and will not alter the qualities of the herbs, interfere with chemical reactions, or be damaged by the corrosive nature of some essential oils or vinegar the way plastic, aluminum, cast iron, and other metals might be.

CLEANING

A colander and a salad spinner are handy for washing any fresh herbs that need to be cleaned. You may have to clean roots with a stiff vegetable brush, or if the skin is particularly tough, with a vegetable parer.

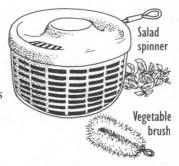

Salad spinner

Vegetable brush

GRINDING

A mortar and pestle are useful for bruising seeds or grinding small quantities of herbs. A small electric coffee grinder works well, but use it solely for herbs. Pulverize dried herbs by rubbing them between your hands, or place large quantities in a pillowcase or locking plastic bag, and roll over them with a rolling pin until they're crushed.

Crush herbs in a pillowcase.

Wood vs. Plastic

Microbiologists at the University of Wisconsin Food Research Institute at Madison discovered that wood cutting boards are naturally better than plastic ones. Plastic encourages bacterial growth, while the porous nature of the wood pulls moisture from microorganisms, causing their rapid death. Although plastics are now made with antibiotics added, experts feel they contribute to the alarming speed with which microorganisms are becoming immune to antibiotics. To prevent bacterial contamination, wash all cutting boards in hot soapy water after each use. Rinse. Sprinkle with baking soda, then spray with herbal vinegar. Let stand 10 minutes. Rinse again, and dry thoroughly.

CUTTING, CHOPPING, AND GRATING

I often use a sharp knife and a hardwood cutting board that I reserve only for herb chopping. You can also use scissors to cut up some herbs, or a food processor to mince herbs and to grate roots. For small quantities, you can use a standard, four-sided hand grater.

MEASURING

It's helpful to have a selection of glass and stainless-steel measuring cups and spoons in different sizes. If you intend to do a lot of work with essential oils, you may want to get a milliliter measure, or several glass eyedroppers. A scale that can weigh in ounces and grams is essential for some formulas.

Safety first. Always wear gloves when weighing or measuring potentially irritating or sensitizing ingredients like essentials oils, borax, washing soda, and ammonia.

Electronic scale, measuring tools, and rubber gloves

MIXING

Sometimes a blender is useful for mixing liquids, but powders and dry ingredients should be mixed in a bowl. A selection of Pyrex or Corelle bowls of various sizes may be the most useful items in my kitchen. For large quantities, I've been known to use my biggest stainless-steel pot. Depending upon the size of the batch, you may need to use various-sized stainless-steel utensils, from teaspoons to serving spoons.

Safety first. When working with powdered ingredients, wear a dust mask to protect mucous membranes. Masks are inexpensive, and readily available at hardware and paint stores.

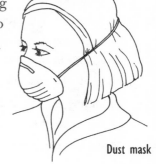

Dust mask

HEATING

I use a whistling stainless-steel teakettle to heat water, but an enameled one would be okay, too. Thermometers are essential if you're making formulas for wood and leather moisturizing and polishing creams. Double boilers are needed for formulas that use wax.

Teakettle and thermometers

AGING

Some formulas, and most herbal extractions (except infusions, page 19, and decoctions, page 20), require a steeping or aging period. This is done in wide-mouthed glass jars with sealing lids. I keep several dozen pint, quart, half-gallon, and gallon jars for this purpose.

STRAINING

Herbal extractions should be strained before use. I usually just pour small batches through a stainless-steel tea strainer. Large batches go in a yogurt strainer, made of fine-meshed fabric, placed inside a glass measuring cup. Some herbalists strain through layers of muslin, either suspended like a jelly bag or tied over a bowl.

Straining separates most of the solids from the liquid. Perfectionists will want to filter the strained liquid, using an unbleached or oxygen-bleached coffee filter. I almost always skip this step for household formulas. I think it's just extra work, but if you strain through a coarse strainer, you may need to filter.

Straining equipment

STORING

I use stainless-steel funnels to transfer mixtures to storage containers: a narrow-tipped one for liquids and a wide-mouthed canning funnel for powdered and dry blends. I store liquids in various-sized amber glass bottles. The color blocks light that would degrade the contents. I use wide-mouthed glass pint jars for waxes and polishes. Powdered formulas can be kept in wide-mouthed jars or tins with a tight seal but should be put in small shaker jars, such as Parmesan cheese containers, for use.

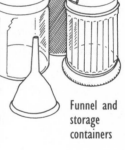

Funnel and storage containers

LABELING

Once your herbal cleaning supplies are packaged, label and date them. Sometimes I run off labels on my laser printer, but a permanent marker or china pencil will work well, too. The important thing is to make sure no one uses floor polish as a medicinal ointment, or drinks toilet cleaner thinking it's an herbal elixir.

MISCELLANEOUS EQUIPMENT

A few more items come in handy, such as candy molds, mini-muffin pans, or butter or cookie molds for casting beeswax. I've made a hobby over the years of collecting kitchen items from estate sales, outlet stores, and catalogs.

BASIC INGREDIENTS

Many herbal cleaning formulas are based on a few simple techniques, which you'll learn about later in this chapter. But before I show you how to proceed with techniques, you need a bit of information about some common ingredients that you'll use over and over again when you begin to make your own housekeeping products: alcohol, ammonia, essential oils, fixatives, fixed oils, glycerin, vinegar, and, most basic of all, water. Many other ingredients appear in the recipes, and on page 136 you'll find a chart, Herbal Housekeeping Ingredients, that describes each one, and tells you its uses and where to get it.

Alcohol. Alcohol is a clear, colorless, volatile, flammable liquid. Both essential oils and water mix with alcohol, making alcohol a necessity for formulas requiring the cleaning power or fragrance of essential oils, since essential oils don't mix with water. You can also use alcohol to extract chemicals from both fresh and dried herbs.

Grain alcohol, also called ethyl alcohol, is derived from yeast fermentation of grain and is sold at liquor stores. Ask for 190-proof alcohol, which is 95 percent alcohol. I feel it's the safest alcohol to use for household formulas.

Denatured alcohol is sold at paint stores for about a third of the price of grain alcohol. A poisonous substance is added to it to make it unfit for human consumption, but it is still suitable for other purposes.

Isopropyl alcohol is made from propylene. Commonly known as rubbing alcohol, it's sold at pharmacies. It is more toxic than grain alcohol and less toxic than denatured alcohol, but is sold for external use only. It costs about the same as denatured alcohol.

In my cleaning formulas, I specify a particular type of alcohol, and also whether any substitutions are allowable. Let your budget be your guide. Whatever type of alcohol you use, be sure to clearly label NOT INTENDED FOR HUMAN

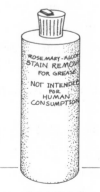

Label all home-made products.

Testing for Allergic Reactions

It's important to understand how to test for allergic reactions before getting into a cleaning solution up to your elbows. Always do a patch test for every new ingredient in any formula to which your skin will be exposed. Apply the substance as described below, cover with an adhesive bandage, then check in 24 hours. If your skin is raised, bumpy, red, raw, irritated, oozing, or otherwise damaged, do not use the ingredient, or wear gloves when working with it.

For liquid materials. To test strong herb tea infusions and decoctions and diluted soaps, or fixed oils like olive, almond, sesame, hazelnut, canola, and safflower, apply a few drops to the inside of your forearm.

For essential oils. Place 1 drop oil into a teaspoon of a fixed oil, such as olive, walnut, mineral, or jojoba, that you know is safe for use on your skin. Apply a little to the inside of your forearm.

For dry materials. If you're working with dry materials like powdered roses and arrowroot starch, dissolve them in a small amount of water (enough to make a paste), and apply to the inside of your forearm.

CONSUMPTION. Call a Poison Control Center immediately if you suspect that anyone has ingested household cleaning formulas containing nonpotable alcohol.

Ammonia. A diluted solution of ammonium hydroxide, ammonia is a clear liquid with a pungent, penetrating odor. It has many cleaning and laundry applications because it is especially good at cutting grease and cleaning woolens. The fumes are unpleasant, and I clean with ammonia solutions only when I have a really heavy-duty cleaning chore and can ventilate the room by opening doors and windows.

Safety first. Never combine ammonia with bleach or a product containing bleach. A chemical reaction occurs that releases potentially toxic fumes. Cleaning formulas made with ammonia should be clearly labeled NOT INTENDED FOR HUMAN CONSUMPTION.

Essential oils. Essential oils are concentrated volatile compounds that are commercially steam-distilled or pressed from aromatic plant material. To understand how concentrated these oils are, note that herbs rarely contain more than 2 percent (and often less than 0.5 percent) of their essential oil. Oils can easily be mixed with alcohol, and in some cases, with glycerine. Oils that are solvent-extracted are called absolutes and may contain small amounts of the solvent used. Purchase essential oils and absolutes from a local health food store or mail-order supplier.

The chart on pages 140–41 lists 21 popular essential oils; following that is a chart that includes essential oils with fixative properties. Besides those, many other essential oils are good for personal and household aromatherapeutic uses: bergamot, black pepper, chamomile, geranium, hyssop, jasmine absolute, juniper berry, laurel leaf, lemon eucalyptus, myrrh, neroli (orange blossom), niaouli, petitgrain (orange leaf and twig), red thyme, rose absolute, sandalwood, vanilla oleoresin, white thyme, and ylang-ylang. Some are especially effective disinfectants. Thyme oil, for instance, contains thymol, which is more powerful than phenol, the chemical used to clean hospitals.

Safety first. Never take essential oils internally.

Storing Essential Oils

When essential oils age, oxidation occurs, rendering them more likely to cause skin sensitization and less capable of antibacterial activity and immune-system enhancement. In *Essential Oil Safety: A Guide for Health Professionals,* Robert Tisserand and Tony Balacs recommend that essential oils be stored in amber glass bottles and used within six months to one year of opening. Pine and citrus oils degrade the most quickly, as early as six months after the bottle is first opened. To double their life, store all oils in the refrigerator. Be sure that everyone in your household understands that they should not be ingested or handled undiluted. If you have young children, keep oils in a locked cupboard, drawer, or toolbox.

Fixatives can improve all the scented formulas in this book. These fragrant roots, seeds, and resins, as well as some animal-derived materials, possess the special ability to blend the other fragrances in a mixture into a new scent, then to release that scent in a slow, controlled manner. Violet-scented orrisroot, the dried, aged rhizome of Florentine iris, is a favorite of potpourri makers, but many other plants have fixative properties as well. Fixatives have interesting, sometimes strong, even peculiar scents of their own, along with their capacity to blend.

You can grow your own, or purchase dried botanicals, essential oils, or absolutes. Work them into every scented product you create, to make the fragrances linger longer, and to take the edge off harsh or disparate fragrances. You'll find a chart beginning on page 142 that lists 29 useful fixatives.

Florentine iris

Fixed oils are nonvolatile vegetable or animal oils. I recommend linseed, olive, walnut, mineral, and jojoba oils. Find linseed oil at paint, hardware, and home center stores; purchase edible oils at health food and grocery stores or from a mail-order supplier.

Glycerin is a clear, odorless, sweet-tasting, viscous alcohol that is a by-product when animal or vegetable fats and oils are made into soap. It's useful for both extracting and preserving herbal products. Since essential oils mix with it, and it mixes with liquid soaps, it also serves as a vehicle for adding fragrance to manufactured soap products. You can buy glycerin at pharmacies, health food stores, and from mail-order suppliers.

Vinegar is a dilute acetic acid made by fermenting grains or fruits. When it has been distilled to remove the brown color, it's labeled as distilled white vinegar. It's available at grocery stores; stock up when it's on sale.

Water is wonderful stuff! The water used in these formulas should be filtered, if at all possible. If not, well water is preferable to distilled water. Get it from your tap or buy it at the grocery store. I use double-filtered tap water.

Safety First Guidelines

- Pay attention to use restrictions and safety information in this book and on the containers of any raw ingredients incorporated into your cleaning products.

- Allergy-test any ingredients that your skin will be exposed to (see Testing for Allergic Reactions on page 13), and if you are prone to allergic reactions, test all ingredients before working with them.

- Always wear gloves when working with undiluted essential oils, strong soap solutions, minerals like washing soda, and chemicals like ammonia.

- If you spill undiluted essential oil on your skin, dilute it immediately with any fixed oil before attempting to wash it off.

- Always wear a dust mask when working with powdered ingredients.

- Always ensure adequate ventilation when working with essential oils, ammonia, and other strongly scented products.

- Never mix any product containing bleach with any product containing ammonia, as the combination produces noxious fumes.

- Label all cleaning products with a complete list of all ingredients and any cautions.

- Keep the local Poison Control Center phone number written in a handy place.

- Store all potentially dangerous ingredients and products in places that children and pets cannot get into, just as you would with any other cleaning supplies. A locked cupboard is best.

- Store any flammable products and ingredients, like waxes, alcohols, and solvents, in glass or metal containers away from heat and open flames.

- Carefully dispose of flammable rags impregnated with waxes or solvents.

- Keep a fire extinguisher (or a large box of baking soda) in your kitchen, garage, and basement.

Herbal Housekeeping Formulas

Although I make many "simples" (the term for formulas that use only one herb), I most enjoy making compounds, which require multiple herbs. Not only do herbal compounds create unique fragrances, but they also allow you to use more than one herb to fight particular organisms like staph, strep, and herpes.

Using dried herbs makes it possible to combine plants that peak at different times of the year, and purchasing herbs lets you use herbs that require different growing conditions than you can provide in your garden. But you can also let your herb garden guide your choice. Each week something new peaks in the garden, so I tend to go out, basket in hand, to collect whatever is there. During the garden season, my formulas are composed of fresh herbs that are at their best at the same time. In the spring, lady's mantle blooms beautifully, providing a lightly scented, mildly astringent solution good for surface cleaning. After that, the roses, lavender, and lemon thyme come into their own. Later in the summer fennel, mints, and coneflowers are ready at the same time, so I combine these herbs for a solution with a sweet scent and an enlivening and antiseptic effect.

Gather fresh herbs in a shallow basket.

USING HERBS SAFELY

Many herbs and essential oils that are powerful antiseptic disinfectants or insect repellents have components that range from very mildly toxic to seriously toxic if they are ingested as a concentrated essential oil. But most — even those with dangerous components — are quite safe when used in extract form in cleaning solutions, or I wouldn't use them. I provide safety information wherever appropriate because I want to help you decide whether to use a particular herb or essential oil or to select another, safer one, even if the alternate choices might be less effective. For instance, if you are expecting a child, you should work only with the safest, least toxic materials. Formulations for cleaning a baby's room should be made with safe herbs like lavender, roses, chamomile, and spearmint, rather than the stronger wormwood, southernwood, tansy, and rue.

In any case, it's important that you label all herbal housecleaning solutions clearly. Make sure that the label clearly indicates the name of the product, its use, a list of its ingredients, and the warning that it is not food. Stored in the refrigerator or kitchen cabinet without a label, herbal housekeeping products can easily be mistaken for something edible.

THE BASIC FORMULAS

The basic method for making an herbal extraction is simple: you combine finely chopped fresh or dried herb with a liquid. Making housekeeping recipes doesn't require the exactitude you might aim for when you're making an extraction for medicinal use. I make them using the folk method, which requires no weighing or measuring. Everything goes much faster that way, and I achieve perfectly satisfactory results with the least amount of effort.

Mixing. I harvest fresh herbs, flowers, or other plant materials in the morning, then chop or cut the plant material with a knife or scissors. If you're using dried material, either purchased or your own stored herbs, crumble them between your hands. Use a mortar and pestle to bruise seeds and crush roots. If you buy herbs for this purpose, buy them in a cut and sifted form whenever possible, rather than whole or powdered.

Fill jars at least three-quarters full if herbs are fresh, leaving at least an inch clearance at the top. The finer you chop the herbs, the lower their level should be in the jar. If you're using dried herbs, fill the jar only halfway. Add the liquid as described on the following pages.

Fill jar ¾ full with fresh herbs for an extraction.

A Jar of Herbs

For all extractions, use a wide-mouthed glass jar with a lid that seals tightly. Don't use a two-piece lid, because it will leak as you shake the jar. Solutions containing vinegar should be sealed with plastic rather than metal lids, as the vinegar reacts with metal.

Storing. Herbal solutions made with water are intended for immediate use. Keep solutions made with other solvents in a cool dark place, shake or stir them daily, and allow them to steep for about 10 days, until the liquid extracts the virtues of the herbs — that is, the chemicals soluble in that particular liquid. You can use the extracted herbal solution either directly or blended first with other ingredients, like soap.

The basic recipes that follow describe the various ways to make herbal extractions, such as solar infusions and decoctions. When you follow one of the specific cleaning formula recipes in Chapter 5, it will specify what type of extraction you need to start with.

Infusions

An infusion is created by steeping herbs in water to release the herbs' water-soluble components. Because herbal solutions for cleaning should be strong, you'll need much larger quantities for a cleaning infusion than you would to make a tea for drinking. The amounts given on page 20 assume that you'll be using a quart jar to make your infusion. Adjust all amounts if you use a different-sized container. Be sure the container you use is heat-proof. My favorite piece of equipment for making infusions and decoctions is an old Pyrex coffeepot with a lid. The spout makes it easy to pour the liquid through a strainer.

Cold infusions are not recommended for housework, as they allow for continued breeding of any bacteria or other microscopic life forms on the herbs.

BASIC METHOD FOR MAKING AN INFUSION

1. Place herbs in a container.
2. Boil water, and pour it over the herbs, filling the container to within an inch or two of the top. Stir rapidly with a stainless-steel spoon or fork, just to be sure the herbs are fully saturated. Put on the lid and allow to steep for at least 15 minutes.
3. Strain and use immediately while the infusion is still hot, especially if you're planning to add soap. Otherwise, refrigerate it for use within a few days. To use later, heat it up on the stove or in the microwave oven, but do not bring to a boil.

2 cups dried herb flowers and/or leaves, crumbled (3 cups fresh, chopped)

3–3½ cups water

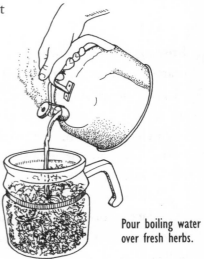

Pour boiling water over fresh herbs.

Decoctions

A decoction is created by simmering tougher plant materials, such as roots, barks, seeds, peels, and fruits, to release the chemicals from the plants.

BASIC METHOD FOR MAKING A DECOCTION

1. Place fresh plant material and 3 cups of water in a heat-proof container, and bring to a simmer. (With dried material, use 5 cups of water. You can double or triple these amounts, proportionally, if desired.)

What You Need

1 cup roots, barks, seeds, peels, or fruits

3–5 cups water

2. Simmer until the water is reduced by half. Keep an eye on the pot, and do not allow the water to evaporate too much. Scorched herbs smell awful!

3. Strain and use the decoction immediately while it's still hot, especially if you're planning to add soap. Otherwise, refrigerate it and use it within a few days. To use later, reheat it on the stove or in the microwave.

Add herbs and simmer until water reduces by half.

Decoction-Infusion Combination

This method works well when you want to combine delicate materials like mint, which cannot tolerate boiling, with something tougher, like pine bark, that requires boiling.

BASIC METHOD FOR MAKING A DECOCTION-INFUSION COMBINATION

What You Need
1 cup roots, barks, seeds, peels, or fruits
1 cup flowers and/or leaves
3–5 cups water

1. Place roots, barks, seeds, peels, or fruits and 3 cups of water in a heat-proof container, and bring the mixture to a simmer. (With dried plant material, use 5 cups of water.)

2. Simmer until the water is reduced by half. Watch carefully and do not allow water to evaporate too much.

3. Remove from heat. Add delicate leaves and flowers. Stir well. Add additional hot water, if necessary.

4. Cover and allow to steep for at least 15 minutes.

5. Strain and use immediately while the mixture is still hot, especially if you're planning to add soap. Otherwise, refrigerate it for use within a few days. To use later, reheat it on the stove or in the microwave oven, but do not boil.

Vinegar Extraction

I make more herbal cleaning solutions with vinegar than with any other solvent. Be sure each jar has a tightly sealed, nonmetal lid that won't react with the vinegar. You can purchase inexpensive plastic lids that fit standard-sized canning jars. The amounts given here assume that you'll be using a quart jar to make your extraction.

If you're in a hurry, you can speed the process by heating the vinegar and pouring the hot vinegar onto the herbs. You can simply steep for at least 15 minutes, then strain and use, but it is better to allow the herbs to steep in the vinegar for at least a few days.

BASIC METHOD FOR MAKING A VINEGAR EXTRACTION

What You Need
2 cups dried herb flowers and/or leaves, crumbled (3 cups fresh, chopped)
3–3½ cups vinegar

1. Place herbs in jar.
2. Fill the jar with vinegar. Be sure all herbs are covered completely. Use a stainless-steel fork or spoon to press down the herbs into the liquid if necessary. Tighten the lid and shake the jar.
3. Put the jar in a cool, dark place for about 10 days. Check it within the first 24 hours and add more vinegar if herbs have swelled above the level of the liquid. Shake occasionally.
4. After 10 days, strain into a narrow-mouthed bottle. Label, and use as needed.

Alcohol Extraction

Because you are using potable grain alcohol, isopropyl alcohol, or denatured grain alcohol, never heat this mixture, as it can spontaneously combust or explode. (See pages 12–13 for information about alcohol types and their uses.) The amounts given on the following page assume that you will be using a quart jar to make your extraction. If your container is a different size, adjust the recipe proportionally.

BASIC METHOD FOR MAKING AN ALCOHOL EXTRACTION

1. Place herbs in jar.
2. Fill the jar with alcohol. Be sure all herbs are covered completely. Use a stainless-steel fork or spoon to press down the herbs into the liquid if necessary. Tighten the lid and shake the jar.
3. Put the jar in a cool, dark place for about 10 days. Check it within 24 hours and add more alcohol if herbs have swelled above the level of the liquid. Shake occasionally.
4. After 10 days, strain into a narrow-mouthed bottle. Label, and use as needed.

What You Need

2 cups dried herb flowers and/or leaves (3 cups fresh)

3–3½ cups alcohol

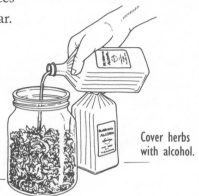

Cover herbs with alcohol.

Ammonia Extraction

Do not heat ammonia on the stove; its fumes are too intense. The amounts given here assume that you're using a quart jar for your extraction; adjust them proportionally if you use a different-sized container.

BASIC METHOD FOR MAKING AN AMMONIA EXTRACTION

1. Place herbs in jar.
2. Fill the jar with ammonia. Be sure all herbs are covered completely. Use a stainless-steel fork or spoon to press down the herbs into the liquid if necessary. Tighten the lid and shake the jar.

What You Need

2 cups dried herb flowers and/or leaves (3 cups fresh)

3–3½ cups ammonia

3. Put the jar in a cool, dark place for about 10 days. Check it within 24 hours and add more ammonia if herbs have swelled above the level of the liquid. Shake occasionally.
4. Strain into a narrow-mouthed bottle. Label, and use as needed.

Glycerin Extraction (Glycerates)

Glycerin will extract more herbal components if you dilute it with 190-proof alcohol, at a rate of 1 part alcohol to 10 parts glycerin (1 tablespoon plus 2 teaspoons of alcohol per cup of glycerin). If you plan to use this solution as a soak to restore flexibility to brittle plastic containers or vinyl shower curtains, however, don't dilute the glycerin with alcohol. The amounts given here assume that you're using a quart jar for the extraction.

BASIC METHOD FOR MAKING A GLYCERIN EXTRACTION

1. Place herbs in jar.
2. Fill the jar with glycerin. Be sure all herbs are covered completely. Use a stainless-steel fork or spoon to press down the herbs into the liquid if necessary. Tighten the lid and shake the jar.
3. Put the jar in a cool, dark place for about 10 days. Check it within the first 24 hours and add more glycerin if herbs have swelled above the level of the liquid. Shake occasionally.
4. After 10 days, strain the mixture into a narrow-mouthed bottle. Label, and use as needed.

What You Need

1 cup dried herb flowers and/or leaves (3 cups fresh)

3–3½ cups glycerin

Quality Control

How can you judge the quality of an herbal extract? As much as possible, it should smell recognizably of the fresh or dried herbs in it, combined with the scent of the extract agent, when vinegar, ethyl alcohol, glycerin, or oil is used. You shouldn't detect off odors, rankness, rot, or rancidity. (The exceptions are herbs extracted in ammonia or isopropyl alcohol; both have such a pungent scent that it's very difficult to smell the herbs in them.)

Oil Extraction (Infused Oil)

Homemade infused oils are extractions created by saturating plant material in a nonvolatile oil in order to withdraw all the oil-soluble components. They are very different from essential oils, which are concentrated compounds produced under lab conditions (see page 14). To make infused oils, use powdered or pulverized dried herbs. Because fresh herbs contain water, they tend to turn the herbal oil rancid.

Infused oils probably require the most work of any herbal extraction method. Straining is a particular challenge. The particles must be removed completely to avoid bacterial contamination. You can let the herbal residue ("marc") settle and then siphon off the oil using tubing, or you can strain the solution. The more traditional method below is followed by a shortcut process on page 26.

BASIC METHOD FOR MAKING INFUSED OIL

1. Put the herbs in a wide-mouthed jar.
2. Add the oils, stirring carefully. Add enough oil so that the herbs are completely covered and there is ½ inch of oil above the top of the herbs.
3. Tighten the lid, and place the jar in a dark, warm place for 10 days, checking after the first 24 hours and adding more oil if necessary. Shake or stir daily.
4. To siphon off the oil, use clean, clear, ¼-inch plastic tubing (available at home centers). Put one end of the tubing in the jar of infused oil with the herbs. Suck gently on the end of the tube until the oil starts flowing, then thrust the end into a cup placed below the level of the jar.
5. Strain the oil through a fine-mesh tea strainer.

What You Need

2 cups dried herb flowers and/or leaves

About 3 cups oil (mineral, olive, or jojoba)

¾ teaspoon vitamin E oil (to prevent rancidity)

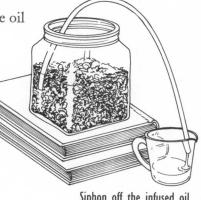

Siphon off the infused oil into a vessel placed at a lower level.

SHORTCUT METHOD FOR MAKING INFUSED OIL

1. Combine the herbs and oil in the top of a double boiler.
2. Heat to 100°F, and maintain this temperature for 6 hours. Allow to cool.
3. Strain into a glass jar. Add the vitamin E oil. Use immediately.

What You Need

1 cup powdered dried herbs
1 cup oil (mineral, olive, or jojoba)
¼ teaspoon vitamin E oil

Dark, Warm Storage Areas

Herbalists sometimes have to be creative to find warm spots in which to make their infused oils. Some place the jars in brown paper bags and leave them in the sun for 10 days; others I know bury their jars in a sandbox. Some put them on top of their refrigerator, while others use a heating pad or an electric yogurt maker to create a consistently warm environment.

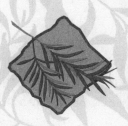

CHAPTER 3

HOUSEKEEPING
Herbs A to Z

O nce you begin to grow your own herbs and learn to recognize their textures, fragrances, and many uses, you'll quickly come to have your own favorites. For this chapter, I've selected 34 easy-to-grow herbs that I have enjoyed growing at one time or another over the past 20 years. I've also chosen plants that have a long tradition of use and, whenever possible, herbs for which there is contemporary research verifying their uses as housekeeping herbs. All of these herbs are available in bulk from health food stores or suppliers, so it's possible for you to purchase plants and dried botanicals that you don't grow in your garden but need for the housekeeping recipes. The chapter concludes with a chart designed to guide you to the recipes that will help you with each of your housekeeping tasks.

ANISE *Pimpinella anisum*

Also known as: Aniseed
Plant type: Annual

The Greek philosopher Theophrastus (about 372–287 B.C.) promoted placing anise by the bedside to prevent bad dreams. In modern aromatherapy, anise is used to alleviate stress, ease relaxation, and aid in establishing healthy sleep patterns. Theophrastus was on the right track!

Uses. Anise is a sweetly scented antiseptic that can be used in sachet bags, potpourris, air fresheners, sweet washing and rinsing waters, and for mousetrap bait when mixed with peanut butter. Extract it in water, vinegar, alcohol, or ammonia.

In the garden. This annual plant has lacy, delightfully fragrant leaves. Anise grows from 12 to 24 inches high. It requires a long growing season (120 to 140 days) to produce its tiny, oval, flattened seeds, which contain most of the plant's essential oils. The seeds store well. Sow anise directly in your garden. Thin seedlings to 8 inches apart. Provide wind protection, or grow it among other plants. Carefully hand-weed or smother weeds with mulch, because anise can't handle competition. Provide even moisture during the growing season.

Harvesting. Early in the season, harvest leaves and flowers for use in extracts. After that, leave flowers on plants to develop seeds. For best

Anise

Rely on Your Senses

When you select plants for housekeeping purposes, remember that the fragrance of each plant can often guide you to its appropriate use. For instance, pungently aromatic, bitter herbs, like wormwood, are often insect chasers. Sweetly scented plants, like lavender, may be antiseptic. Astringent herbs, like yarrow, usually contain tannins — chemicals that may dry up the cell walls of bacteria.

For housekeeping purposes, select sweetly aromatic or pungently scented herbs and bitter, astringent, or sour-tasting plants from those native to your region, and experiment with water, vinegar, alcohol, and ammonia extractions to discover their properties. Often herbs with a tradition of medical use also make good housekeeping herbs. These include chamomile, thyme, rosemary, sage, and lavender. If plants suggested in the formulas don't grow in your climate and soil conditions, ask your local Extension Service office, Herb Society of America branch, or garden club which useful plants you can grow in their places.

yields, harvest green, fully formed seeds and ripen them indoors by hanging several bundled stems upside down inside a brown paper bag or over a clean cloth that will catch them as they drop. When seeds are fully dried, shake them or rub them away from their stems. Store in a cool, dark place in sealed tins or glass jars. Use some for formulas, and some to start next year's plants.

ANISE HYSSOP *Agastache foeniculum*
Also known as: Licorice mint, lavender mint
Plant type: Hardy perennial

Native Americans used anise hyssop as a medicinal plant, and enjoyed it as a tea. The Cheyenne Indians used it in perfumes. The entire plant is strongly, sweetly aromatic. Its licorice scent reminds me of old-fashioned, hard black candies, dusted with powdered sugar. Bees love it!

Anise Hyssop

Uses. Collected when newly opened, the flowers dry well for potpourri and wreaths. Use leaves and flowers in sweet washing waters, simmering potpourri, and herb decorations. Extract it in water, vinegar, alcohol, or ammonia.

In the garden. Anise hyssop is a hardy perennial, with the typical square stems of a mint; it self-sows readily. Growing 3 to 4 feet tall, it has purplish stems and dark green leaves. Small edible flowers are a lovely pinkish purple and rise up from the plant like cathedral spires, 2 to 6 inches long. Grow anise hyssop from seed sown in spring or autumn, or buy plants. Space 2 feet apart, in full sun or dappled shade. Pinch back to encourage branching. *Zones 4-9.*

Harvesting. Harvest snippets from midsummer onward, but leave at least a third of the plant to grow, except in late autumn, when all the above-ground parts of the plant can be harvested. Use it fresh or dried.

BASIL *Ocimum basilicum*

Also known as: Sweet basil (cultivars are identified by scent, such as cinnamon basil and lemon basil)
Plant type: Tender perennial (treated as an annual)

Basil has a reputation for inciting strong passions of both love and hatred, and literature is full of allusions to its powers. In Hindu herbalism and spiritual practices, it is considered to open the heart and mind, making possible a feeling of great spiritual love and devotion. Its fragrance is spicy, warm, rich, and aromatic.

Basil

Uses. Basil is antiseptic and antibacterial, and mildly enhances the immune system. It is a powerful surface and air cleanser. Extract it in water, vinegar, alcohol, or ammonia.

In the garden. Basil grows to 2 feet, with 2- to 3-inch-long oval, green leaves with toothed edges. Cultivars like 'Lettuce Leaved' and 'Ruffles' have slightly crumpled leaves. To get a head start on the season in northern regions, start seed indoors four to six weeks before the last spring frost. As basil grows, pinch off the second or third set of leaves on each new stem, and soon you will have a very large, bushy plant. To prevent bloom, pinch off buds by pinching the stem back to the next set of leaves below the buds.

Basil requires a well-drained soil, rich in nitrogen and high in organic matter in full sun. It will grow in just about any pH — 5.0 to 8.0. But, it cannot withstand even a light frost, so harvest the whole plant when cold weather threatens.

Harvesting. Collect snippets all summer long, then harvest the whole plant before frost threatens. Use the chopped plant fresh in water, vinegar, and alcohol extracts, or hang bunches to dry in a cool, dark place.

SACRED BASIL *Ocimum tenuiflorum*

Also known as: Holy basil, tulasi, tulsi
Plant type: Tender perennial (treated as an annual)

Much valued in India, sacred basil is often grown around temples for use in religious ceremonies. An infusion of the leaves in water may be sprinkled on worshipers, or foods flavored with tulsi may be offered to them. Hindus make beads of the wooden stems of the older plants, then string them into *malas,* which they use as rosaries to keep track of the number of prayers or chants uttered, as well as to protect them against disease.

Sacred
Basil

Uses. Sacred basil's sweet fragrance makes it a natural for potpourri, simmering potpourri, and sachets. The flower spikes make lovely accents in wreaths, ornaments, and everlasting arrangements. Its refreshing and cleansing characteristics make it suitable for use in water, vinegar, and alcohol extractions. It is sometimes used to repel mosquitoes.

In the garden. Sacred basil has hairy leaves, shorter, smaller, rounder, and less puckered than those of sweet basil. The flowers are pink or purple, and the fragrance is sweeter and less pungent. Provide as for sweet basil. Sacred basil can be successfully grown as a container plant. Of all the basils, this is the one most likely to self-sow if you let it bloom and set seed. Or, propagate it from cuttings.

Harvesting. Same methods as for sweet basil.

CAMPHOR BASIL
Ocimum kilimandscharicum
Also known as: Feverplant
Plant type: Tender perennial (treated as an annual)

During World War II, camphor basil provided an alternative source of camphor, used to repel insects. This is valued as a medical, rather than a culinary, herb. Its strong camphor scent is distinctive.

Uses. The same compounds that give camphor basil its medicinal power also make it useful for cleaning, disinfecting, and repelling insects, especially moths and mosquitoes.

Camphor Basil

In the garden. Camphor basil's leaves are longer and narrower than those of sweet basil, and they have a coating of fine hairs. The flowers are white. Provide the same conditions as you would for sweet basil, although in Park's *Success with Herbs,* Gertrude B. Foster and Rosemary F. Loudon recommend cooler night temperatures (55°F) for germination. It can also be propagated from cuttings.

Harvesting. Treat as you would sweet basil.

BAY *Laurus nobilis*
Also known as: Bay laurel, sweet bay, green bay, Grecian bay, Roman bay
Plant type: Evergreen tree

Sacred to the sun god Apollo, whose temple was built in a grove of bay trees, bay was thought to protect one from all harm, including lightning strikes and epilepsy, and impart virtue. In ancient Greece and Rome, it was used to crown emperors, honored statesmen, esteemed poets, admired philosophers, and victorious athletes.

Bay

Safety first. *While bay laurel is safe, other plants called laurel, like the American native mountain laurel* (Kalmia latifolia), *are poisonous.*

Uses: Bay is an antibacterial herb and a fungicide. It has many uses, including dry and simmering potpourri, sachets, air fresheners, and washing waters; it repels cockroaches and other insects. Extract it in water, vinegar, alcohol, or ammonia. Putting whole bay leaves into jars of stored grains and beans prevents the eggs of weevils from hatching.
In the garden. This 40- to 60-foot, smooth-barked evergreen tree has a spread of 30 feet, but when grown in a container it usually reaches only about 6 feet. Bay has pointed, tough, shiny, dark green leaves. Its small, greenish yellow flowers bloom in June and July. Mature plants produce blackish purple berries about ½ inch in diameter. Grow bay as a container plant in colder climates so that you can winter it indoors. You can propagate bay by taking 4-inch, semi-hardwood cuttings in autumn, but it's notoriously slow to root, so you may prefer to purchase a plant. Potted bays are susceptible to scale and spider mites, so check plants carefully before purchasing. If you live in a warm climate, plant it in a sunny to mostly sunny spot, in good, well-drained soil with a pH of 4.5 to 8.2. *Zones 8–10.*
Harvesting. Harvest a few leaves at a time, and use them fresh or lay them flat to dry. Drying time will vary with your climate, up to two weeks. Leaves are dry when they are brittle enough to snap easily. Store them in glass jars or tins in a cool, dark place.

Bee Balm

BEE BALM *Monarda fistulosa,*
M. citriodora, M. didyma, M. punctata
Also known as: Lemon bee balm, wild bergamot, Oswego tea, prairie bee balm, spotted bee balm
Plant type: Perennial

Monarda didyma is said to be the plant used as a tea substitute after the Boston Tea Party in 1773. The whole plant is aromatic, and the scents of different types range from the lemon of *citriodora* to a peppery citrus fragrance like that of the bergamot orange; some smell like a combination of oregano and mint.

Uses: Bee balm attracts bees and hummingbirds to the garden. Flowers dry well for arrangements and other crafts, if harvested early. You can use the leaves and flowers in water, vinegar, ammonia, and alcohol extracts for use in insect-repelling recipes. It contains thymol, a powerful antiseptic component of its essential oil, which may inhibit chickenpox and herpes viruses; it is antibacterial as well.

In the garden. This hardy, dark green perennial grows 4 feet tall. Flowers may be red, pink, lilac, or white. Bee balm is susceptible to powdery mildew, but effects are less if grown in full sun with good air circulation. It germinates easily from seed sown outdoors in the spring. If you purchase plants, smell them first, to determine whether you like their fragrance. Bee balm prefers moist, well-drained loamy soil, pH 5.0 to 7.0. Space every 2 feet, and pinch back to encourage bushiness. Plants bloom beautifully in July and August. *Zones 3–9.*

Harvesting. Harvest up to two-thirds of the above-ground parts of the plant when it's in bud. Later, when the plant has grown back, harvest flowers and take another cutting of the top third of the plant. Hang stems to dry or dry on a rack. Use fresh or dried clippings.

CALAMUS *Acorus calamus, A. americanus*
Also known as: Sweet flag, sweet rush, sweet root, sweet sedge
Plant type: Perennial

Calamus is an insect repellent and a fairly common fixative. *Acorus americanus* is safer than the Asian species, *A. calamus.* It was widely used by Native Americans as food, perfume, and medicine.
Uses. Use calamus in potpourris and sleep pillows, for surface washing and insect chasing, and wherever you need an antiseptic and antibac-terial herb. Extract it in water, vinegar, alcohol, or ammonia. In India, calamus powder is used as a flea and white ant repellent. It sterilizes male grain weevils so they can't reproduce.

Calamus

Safety first. Although it should not be used for food or medicine, calamus is considered safe for housekeeping purposes.

In the garden. This hardy, 2- to 3-foot perennial has long, narrow, sword-shaped leaves that are yellowish green and aromatic when bruised. In June it bears a long, narrow, yellow-green flower that juts out at a 45-degree angle. The fragrant rhizomes have a reddish brown peel and a white interior. Propagate calamus by root division, planting rhizomes about a foot apart, in either spring or autumn in the wettest, marshiest part of the garden. Calamus likes a pH range of 5.0 to 7.5 and prefers some shade, but it will grow in full sun if the roots are in water. (Its natural habitat is wet, marshy areas alongside slow-moving streams, ponds, and lakes.) It seems to grow equally well in sand or clay, but will spread faster in sandy soil. *Zones 3–9.*

Harvesting. Gather the leaves for fresh use at any time, and the rhizomes in the late autumn or early spring when they are at least two and not more than three years old, as they become hollow when they age. Wash roots well, but do not peel them, since the essential oil content is highest in the peel. When they're still fresh, cut them into segments or slices, or grate them. (Dried whole, they send out new leaf shoots, which weaken their power.) Spread them on a drying rack. Dry until brittle, then store in a sealed tin or glass jar in a cool, dark place.

CHAMOMILE *Matricaria recutita*

Also known as: German chamomile
Plant type: Annual

All of the ancient herbalists extolled the use of chamomile for its soothing, healing effects, and considered it safe enough for children. Even Beatrix Potter's much-loved Peter Rabbit was put to bed by his mother with a cup of chamomile tea for his tummy ache. The delicious, fruity fragrance of chamomile is similar to that of apple and pineapple.

German
Chamomile

Uses. Chamomile is a gentle but tough cleaner that is effective against bacteria and fungi, including candida and staph. Its immune-stimulating powers make it a good cleanser. Use leaves and flowers, dried or fresh, in cleaning formulas calling for water, vinegar, alcohol, or ammonia extractions. Place dried flowers in sleep pillows and in potpourris (dried and simmering) for their fruity fragrance.

Safety first. *Tests show that chamomile may cause hayfeverlike symptoms for about 8 out of 100 people who are allergic to ragweed.*

In the garden. A rather scruffy, lanky annual plant, chamomile grows to 2 feet tall. It has feathery leaves, and sunny little white daisy flowers with yellow centers. Sow chamomile directly in the garden; it's difficult to transplant. Chamomile requires full sun, sandy soil, and a pH of 5.0 to 8.0; thin plants to 4 to 6 inches apart. If transplanting larger, purchased plants, be sure to pinch them way back. Otherwise, plants will wilt badly from the shock, and they may not recover. Also pinch back plants throughout the growing season to encourage bushiness, or use scissors to shear plants. Chamomile will self-sow on sandy soils if you don't cut off all the flower heads before they set seed.

Harvesting. Harvest both the flowers and leaves for household use, fresh or dried. Always leave at least a third of the plant at midseason harvests, but in autumn, gather the entire plant before frost.

COSTMARY *Chrysanthemum balsamita*

Also known as: Bible leaf, alecost, balsam herb, sweet Mary

Plant type: Hardy perennial

Costmary's leaves have a sweet fragrance, somewhat reminiscent of anise or licorice combined with camphor and spearmint. One of its common names, "Bible leaf," comes from its use in colonial American times as a bookmark in Bibles and prayer books. Not only did it mark the reader's place, but its scent and taste provided diversion during

Costmary

the hours-long services early settlers attended. But because its essential oil is rich in camphor (72–91 percent), costmary also repels insects.

Uses. Costmary is antiseptic and possibly antiparasitical. Use fresh or dried leaves in water, vinegar, ammonia, or alcohol extractions, or in simmering potpourris. Dried leaves can also be used in wreaths. Some people slip them into books to chase away paper-eating insects.

In the garden. A 2- to 3-foot-tall hardy perennial, costmary has 3-inch-long, narrow, oblong, grayish green leaves with a fine saw-toothed edge and insignificant yellow button flowers in late summer. Purchase a plant, or grow from root divisions. Space about a foot and a half apart. Costmary requires full sun, dry, fertile loam with a pH of 4.0 to 6.0, and an occasional side-dressing of compost. When the center begins to die back, divide the root and replant the divisions. *Zones 4–10.*

Harvesting. Gather leaves throughout the growing season. Since the plant dies back to the root, harvest all of the leaves before they brown in autumn, and hang them or lay them on a rack to dry.

ELECAMPANE *Inula helenium*

Also known as: Elf dock, wild sunflower, velvet dock

Plant type: Perennial

Elecampane

Nicholas Culpeper wrote in his 17th-century herbal that elecampane protected against ills like plague and intestinal parasites. In fact, the candied root was eaten to protect against bad air when traveling by river in London. Later researchers found that one of its components, helenin, is so powerful that a .0001 solution destroys bacteria that cause tuberculosis.

Uses. The fresh root is antiseptic, antifungal, and antibacterial. Use it in surface washes in water, vinegar, ammonia, or alcohol extractions. Wear gloves if you notice any sensitivity.

In the garden. This hardy 4- to 6-foot-tall perennial has an erect stem, and branches only at the top. The oval leaves are large, often close to 1½ feet long and 4 inches across, with a velvety underside. Yellow, daisylike flowers bloom at the top of the plant in June and July. The rootstock is large, with brown skin, a fleshy white interior, and a strong, sweet floral fragrance when fresh, almost superior to that of orrisroot. Elecampane prefers damp ground. It likes full sun, can tolerate dappled shade, handles heavy loam with aplomb, and appreciates a soil pH of 4.5 to 7.4. It propagates easily from seed or from root divisions taken in early spring or autumn. *Zones 2–10.*

Harvesting. Dig up the roots of two-year-old plants in autumn, when the tops have started to die back. Divide the roots and replant some. Scrub clean, peel, grate, and make extracts from the rest.

EPAZOTÉ *Chenopodium ambrosioides*
Also known as: Wormseed, Mexican tea
Plant type: Annual

This entire plant, including its seeds, is scented with a peculiar odor, like many herbs that have the power to destroy intestinal worms. One of its common names refers to this characteristic.

Safety first. The seed oil was formerly used to expel worms and other internal parasites, but is now known to have a depressant action on the heart, making it dangerous to ingest even in small doses. Since the effective dose is so close to the toxic dose, do not use wormseed oil, either internally or externally.

Epazoté

Uses. In the tropics, epazoté is used in a water extract to mop porches and swab down wood posts to deter insects. Use fresh or dried leaves in water, vinegar, ammonia, and alcohol extracts for surface cleaning and bug chasing. Scatter dried leaves on pantry shelves. Grown with container plants, epazoté makes spraying pesticides unnecessary.

In the garden. Some gardeners consider this annual erect plant in the goosefoot family a weed. It can grow to 4 feet but usually goes to seed at half that height, especially if it hasn't had enough water. It has oval leaves, 1 to 3 inches long with a toothed edge, and small yellowish green flowers in July. Sow seed directly in the garden. If any plants are allowed to set seed, they are very likely to self-sow.

Harvesting. Harvest snippings through the season, and collect the whole plant before it goes to seed. Hang to dry.

HYSSOP *Hyssopus officinalis*
Plant type: Perennial

Although *Hyssopus officinalis* is acknowledged for its cleaning powers, the hyssop that the Bible calls a cleansing herb must have been another species, since *H. officinalis* isn't native to the Holy Land. Hyssop has an aromatic scent, reminiscent of pine and camphor. It was one of the strewing herbs, and it's still a useful bee plant.

Hyssop

Uses. Hyssop is an antiviral, antiseptic cleanser and insect chaser used in water, vinegar, ammonia, or alcohol extractions, as well as in sachets. A testimony to its powers, in test-tube research, it acted against both herpes and HIV. Add dried sprigs of leaves and flowers to wreaths and other ornaments.

Safety first. The essential oil of hyssop is much stronger than the plant, and should be avoided by pregnant women and by epileptics who are not on medication.

In the garden. This small (1–2 feet), bushy perennial has narrow, oval, grayish green leaves. A showy display of blue, pink, or white flowers reaches 6 inches above the other stems. Once the flowers have bloomed, clip them off to keep the plant tidy. Propagate from seed, cuttings, or root division. Space plants 1 foot apart in a sunny or mostly sunny position in dry, well-drained soil with a pH of 7.5 to 8.5. When plants are mature, you can divide them in early spring as new growth starts. *Zones 3–8.*

Harvesting. Clip new growth (no more than a third of the plant at a time) two or three times a year. Do not harvest after summer, as the new growth needs time to harden off before cold weather.

LAVENDER *Lavandula angustifolia*
Plant type: Perennial

Lavender was once so highly thought of as a cleansing herb that its name comes from the Latin word *lavare,* meaning "to wash."
Uses. Lavender repels moths and is excellent in sachets, air fresheners, and washing waters. Extract fresh or dried flowers and foliage in water, vinegar, ammonia, or alcohol.
In the garden. A shrubby, multibranched plant, lavender grows about 1½ feet tall and 1½ feet wide, with narrow, 2-inch, grayish green foliage and white, pink- or blue-purple spiky flowers. Propagate from root divisions or cuttings; plants grow slowly from seed. Set plants in full sun, in well-drained, sandy soil with a pH of 6.4 to 8.0. Snip all blooms off the plants during their first year to encourage leafy growth. Spike lavender *(L. latifolia)* and lavandin *(L. × intermedia)* are hardy to Zone 4 and contain more camphor than *L. angustifolia,* making them better moth chasers. *Zones 5–8.*
Harvesting. For bushier plants, harvest 2 inches of foliage early in the season and dry it on a rack. Later, harvest both foliage and flower stems, bundle them, and hang them upside down to dry.

Lavender

LEMON BALM *Melissa officinalis*
Also known as: Sweet balm, balm, Melissa
Plant type: Perennial

Lemon balm has a light, sweet, lemony aroma, with just a hint of aspirin scent. Although its powerful essential oil (sold as Melissa oil) is considered safe, it's quite expensive. Buy it from a reputable supplier that authenticates its oils, as many Melissa oils have been partially or completely "extended" with much cheaper essential oils like lemon and citronella.

Lemon Balm

Uses. Use lemon balm in potpourri, air fresheners, and surface washes. Extract in water, vinegar, alcohol, or ammonia. Antiviral, it's effective against mumps and herpes, and also acts against the flu virus. Although mild, it's a powerful cleaner, and also an antidepressant. And, it's considered safe enough to use around infants.

In the garden. This bushy, rounded perennial herb grows to about 2½ feet high and 1½ feet wide. Its serrated, yellow-green leaves are oval to heart-shaped. It has tiny yellow flower buds that open to inconspicuous white blooms. Propagate lemon balm from seed (it requires light to germinate) or take cuttings or root divisions. Its seeds freely self-sow. Although it likes sun, it can tolerate dappled shade. Set plants in light, fertile, very well-drained soil, with a pH of 4.5 to 7.5. Lemon balm can tolerate drier soil than can many other herbs. *Zones 4–9.*

Harvesting. Harvest sprigs at any time, then when buds form, take about two-thirds of the plant. The fresh leaves make the best extracts, but dried leaves can also be used. Bundle stems and hang them upside down in the dark, if possible, to dry. Lemon balm dries very quickly. Although it blackens as it dries, this does not affect its quality.

MARJORAM *Origanum majorana*

Also known as: Sweet marjoram, knotted marjoram
Plant type: Tender perennial

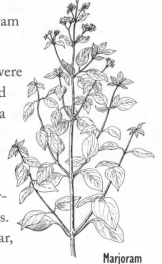

Bridal couples in ancient Greece and Rome were crowned with marjoram because it represented love, honor, and happiness. The whole plant has a delightful aroma, less dry and bitter-smelling than its relative, oregano.

Uses. Fresh marjoram is a nice addition to tussie-mussies and flower arrangements. Use dried marjoram in wreaths, everlastings, and sleep pillows. Use fresh or dried marjoram in water, vinegar, ammonia, or alcohol extracts for surface cleaning.

Marjoram

In the garden. Marjoram is a small, bushy, multistemmed tender perennial, about 1½ feet tall and 1 foot wide. It has small green, rounded leaves, and pink or pinkish white flowers. Aromatic marjoram can be grown from seeds, cuttings, or root divisions. The young plants are prone to damping-off, so try growing in a flat with alternating rows of chamomile. Water the weak, spindly plants from below with chamomile tea; even a gentle shower from above may knock them over. Set out plants in full sun, in dry, preferably sandy, well-drained soil with a pH of 7.0 to 8.0, when the soil has warmed and night temperatures are predictably warm. Space about 6 to 8 inches apart and provide protection from winds and weather. *Zones 8–10.*

Harvesting. Harvest about one third of the plant as it goes into bud. In long growing seasons, you may get another clipping before harvesting the whole plant when frost threatens. Dry in bundles, or use fresh.

MUGWORT *Artemisia vulgaris*
Also known as: St. John's plant
Plant type: Perennial

Mugwort was known to the ancients as the Mother of Herbs. Much lore associates mugwort as a protective herb in Christian and even older rituals. Gathered on St. John's Day (June 24) and made into chaplets to wear and wreaths to hang on doors, in the Middle Ages mugwort was believed to protect against supernatural misfortunes.

Uses. Mugwort is useful in mothproofing blends, as its scent repels wool moths and may prevent the hatching of their eggs, probably due to its camphor content. You can also stuff it in sleep pillows and under mattresses; it's thought to prevent nightmares. Use mugwort as a gray accent in wreaths and everlasting arrangements, and extract it, fresh or dried, in water, vinegar, ammonia, or alcohol to use as a surface cleaner and antiseptic. The dried herb can also be burned as a fumigant.

Mugwort

In the garden. Mugwort is a 4- to 6-foot-tall aromatic perennial, with 2- to 4-inch green leaves whose undersides are downy gray. In July or August, it bears tiny, scruffy gold flowers in grapelike clusters at the ends of the stems. A very hardy perennial, it thrives in full sun and can be easily grown from direct-sown seeds, semi-hardwood cuttings taken in late summer, or root divisions made in early spring or late autumn. Allow the soil to warm before sowing seeds outdoors. Set or thin plants to about a foot or more apart. I shear the early summer growth to encourage branching at the tips of the stems. Mugwort spreads less when the soil is kept a bit dry. *Zones 4–10.*

Appealing Curves

Bundle fine-foliaged plants like mugwort and southernwood, and curve their tips over a cylindrical container (such as an oatmeal box). They'll dry with a lovely curve that adds an elegant touch to floral designs.

Harvesting. Harvest stems by cutting them back by a foot or so in early summer, either before or at the time they bud. Use stems fresh, or bundle and hang them to dry, being careful to smooth leaves downward if you intend to use them in wreaths or arrangements. Take a second cutting of side shoots later in the year, and either use them fresh, or dry them on a rack. Harvest all above-ground parts of the plant in autumn, once plants are mature and growing well.

OREGANO *Origanum heracleoticum*

Also known as: Greek oregano
Plant type: Perennial

One of the most common culinary herbs, oregano can serve many useful housekeeping purposes as well, from antiseptic surface cleaners to fragrant simmering potpourris. The entire plant is aromatic, with a fairly bitter, spicy fragrance.

Uses. Oregano is antiseptic and antiparasitical. Extract it in water, vinegar, ammonia, or alcohol to use in surface washes.

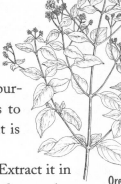

Oregano

Combine oregano with other, sweeter-scented herbs to counter its bitter, pungent fragrance. You can also incorporate the sprigs in wreaths, nosegays, and everlasting arrangements, or use them in potpourri and simmering potpourri in masculine and woody blends.

In the garden. A naturally mound-shaped perennial plant, oregano can reach 1 to 2 feet tall and wide. Its oval leaves are covered with fine hairs. Its white flowers bloom in summer, starting in July. It is best propagated from root divisions or cuttings from a plant whose fragrance you have admired, because there is so much variability in the plants that are grown from seed. If you must grow it from seed, sow a great deal and reject those with substandard scent. To give plants more strength, transplant seedlings at least once after germinating, then plant them outdoors, in full sun, in dry, well-drained soil with a pH of 4.5 to 8.0, after all danger of frost. *Zones 5–10.*

Harvesting. Take sprigs from plants at any time, but harvest heavily as it comes into bud. Allow plants to regrow, and take another cutting from mature plants in late summer. Use oregano fresh or dried, and either hang-dry in bunches or dry it on a rack.

PEPPERMINT *Mentha* x *piperita,* also *M.* x *piperita* var. *citrata*

Also known as: Brandy mint, orangemint
Plant type: Perennial

The ancients wore peppermint in chaplets, garlanded their feasting tables with it, and flavored everything, including wines, with it. Native Americans used mints for medicine before European settlers arrived. Its scent is strong and distinctive — the familiar peppermint of candy and toothpaste. Orangemint, also known as eau de cologne mint, has a bergamot scent that combines orange, lemon, and pepper.

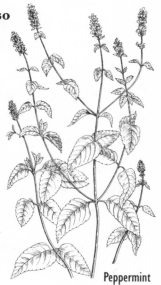

Peppermint

Uses. About half menthol, peppermint oil is antibacterial, antiviral, and antiparasitical. The fresh or dried herb can be used in water, vinegar, ammonia, and alcohol extracts for surface cleaning. It can also be used in potpourri and simmering potpourri, although it will probably have to be refreshed before the rest of the ingredients. The dried flowering tips are very pretty in wreaths and tussie-mussies.

Safety first. *Don't use the essential oil of peppermint in housekeeping recipes if you suffer from cardiac fibrillation.*

In the garden. This hardy 2-foot-tall perennial has dark, round leaves with a toothed edge, square purplish stems, and lilac flowers. These sterile hybrids don't set viable seed. Purchase plants, or obtain runners from existing plants, and space 8 inches apart. Mint flourishes in rich, moist soil with a pH of 7.0 to 8.0 in a sunny to partially shaded area where they'll have room to spread their runners. Harvest older plants and let the younger ones grow. *Zones 3–9.*

Harvesting. Once your mint is established, harvest it freely. You can clip the top third to half of the plants early in the year to encourage branching, then clip again when they're in bloom. Harvest the entire stems of any runners that have gotten out of bounds. You can bundle mint and hang-dry it, or dry it on a rack. When I plan to use flowering tips in flat-backed sprays or swags, I dry them flat.

ROSEMARY *Rosmarinus officinalis*
Plant type: Tender perennial

In the 16th and 17th centuries, rosemary was carried at both weddings and funerals as a symbol of remembrance. Its traditional association with memory seems to have some basis in fact, because its scent does seem to activate the brain. The strong, refreshing, aromatic scent is a combination of eucalyptus, pine, and camphor.

Rosemary

Uses. I love to combine rosemary with lavender to protect clothing from moths. Antiseptic and antiparasitical, the fresh or dried herb can be used in water, vinegar, ammonia, and alcohol extracts for surface cleaning. Add sprigs to wreaths, tussie-mussies, potpourri, simmering potpourri, and sachets. I use essential oil of rosemary as a grease remover. Add the strongly antioxidant essential oil to any formula containing fixed oils to prevent rancidity.

In the garden. In the right climate, this shrubby, tender perennial herb can grow to 6 feet, with a spread of 4 feet. Short, narrow evergreen leaves are dark green above, grayish and finely felted below. Most rosemarys bear blue flowers in December and later, although some cultivars have pink or white flowers. Prostrate and trailing forms make dramatic bonsai. Propagate rosemary from tender cuttings taken in the spring by layering, or purchase a plant. 'Arp' is the only cultivar that withstands cold (to Zone 6), so gardeners in zones colder than 8 usually bring rosemary indoors to winter over. It can be finicky indoors, as it requires high light levels; excellent air circulation; high humidity; rich, well-drained soil (lots of sand and perlite in the mix and frequent applications of compost tea or kelp); and a 20-degree temperature drop at night to be really happy. *Zones 8–10.*

Harvesting. Harvest 2- to 6-inch sprigs from the tips of the branches at any time, being careful not to take more than a quarter (or preferably less) of the length. Use sprigs fresh or dried. Hang-dry or dry them on a rack.

ROSE *Rosa* spp.
Plant type: Shrub

Greek mythology relates that roses get their beauty from Aphrodite; their charm, joy, and brilliance from the three Graces; and their nectar and fragrance from Dionysus. Chloris, the goddess of flowers, declared the rose the queen of flowers, and Aphrodite presented the rose to her son, Eros, god of love, making it

Damask Rose

the symbol of passion — the fusion of love and desire. Flower fragrance varies widely from one species to another, some have hints of anise, lemon, tea, myrrh, musk, or even raspberry.

Uses. Use roses fresh or dried in water, vinegar, and alcohol extractions. They're also wonderful in potpourri, simmering potpourri, sachets, and other crafts. Avoid using them in insect repellents, as they tend to attract many pests. Leave some roses on plants that set hips so that you can collect them for use in extractions, tea, or crafts.

Rosa Gallica
'Versicolor'

In the garden. Long a favorite of gardeners, roses come in shades of white, pink, red, violet, yellow, orange — even bicolored. Some species have pulpy hips containing the seeds. Hips start out green, then turn yellow, orange, and usually ripen red after a frost. Rose species have variable hardiness, so be sure to purchase scented varieties that will grow in your zone.

Roses appreciate rich, well-drained, heavy soil with a pH of 6.5 to 6.8; they may even like a bit of clay. They need full sun to very lightly dappled shade, in a protected area with good air circulation. They should be bottom-watered by a soaker hose to prevent disease. Heavy feeders, roses require side-dressing with compost, kelp, or manure, especially during budding, a time when they also need plenty of water.

To ensure enough roses for household uses, plant several shrubs or climbing roses that bloom over a long period. Roses like being mulched; and in my Zone 5 climate, heavy winter protection in the form of hay, evergreen branches, or leaves is a must. *Zones 3–9.*

Harvesting. Be patient! To encourage robust growth, both roots and above ground, prevent your roses from flowering by religiously plucking all buds for the first two years after you install your plants. (Use the buds in sachets and potpourris.) In the third year, harvest buds and partially opened roses. Use them fresh, or place them on a rack to dry.

SAGE *Salvia officinalis*

Also known as: Garden sage, Dalmatian sage
Plant type: Perennial

Sage is such a powerful antiseptic and digestive stimulant that it was once widely believed that no man with sage in his garden could die — assuming, of course, that he used the sage to make tea and to season foods. Gardens with flourishing sage plants were said to indicate that the wife ruled the household. The French thought it alleviated grief, and in the language of flowers (see page 51), sage stands for health and longevity, along with esteem and domestic virtues. A handy plant to have!

Uses. Sage is antibacterial, antioxidant, and an insect chaser. Use fresh or dried in water, vinegar, ammonia, and alcohol extractions. When combined with rosemary, each is more effective. Hang-dry leaves in bunches for use in culinary wreaths and other everlasting crafts.

Safety first. The essential oil of sage consists of about 50 percent thujone and 26 percent camphor, both of which are toxic. Because of this, Tisserand and Balacs, in Essential Oil Safety, *consider sage essential oil dangerous and recommend against its use in aromatherapy. Pregnant women should avoid the essential oil.*

In the garden. Sage grows to about 2 feet high and just as wide. Gray-green, oval leaves have long stalks and a soft-textured, crinkled surface like a fine velveteen seersucker. Flowers are usually purple, although some cultivars have pink, blue, or white flowers. Sage is easily grown from seed, but if you take cuttings or root divisions in autumn, the plants will mature much faster. Sage prefers full sun, and rich, slightly acidic soil, pH 6.0 to 6.5, with good drainage. *Zones 3–9.*

Harvesting. Snip branches any time after the plant is well established. To increase vegetative growth, prune severely whenever the plant tries to bud. Hang-dry in bundles, or separate leaves and lay them on a rack. After blooming, the dried bracts make interesting everlastings.

SOAPWORT *Saponaria officinalis*

Also known as: Bouncing bet
Plant type: Hardy perennial

Here's a plant with a perfectly suited name. Saponins are suds makers, and the common name, soapwort, means "soap plant." Soapwort was known in the Middle Ages as *herba fullonis,* the "fuller's herb," because it was used to finish wool textiles. "Fulling" is the process of washing woven woolens, which thickens and sometimes felts them.

Uses. The saponins in the root and, to a lesser extent, in the leaves of soapwort are perfect for washing delicate textiles like tapestries. Soapwort is therefore often

Soapwort

used for that purpose by museum curators, as well as herbalists and textile artists. You can extract the root in alcohol, vinegar, or ammonia. If you use ammonia for the extract, soapwort makes a gelatinous mass, which you can use to clean dirty pots, oven racks, and barbecue grills. Coat the surface to be cleaned, allow it to sit overnight, and then rinse. The alcohol extraction is red and should not be used for spot-cleaning nonwashable fabrics.

In the garden. This hardy, deep-green perennial can grow to 2 feet tall on a single hairy stem, which may branch a little at the top. Soapwort is about a foot wide. Its flowers, which bloom July through September, are often pink when in bud, white when newly opened, and pink again when they're fading. Soapwort can be invasive, spreading from the rootstock. It prefers full sun, but will tolerate dappled shade in almost any type of soil with a pH of 6.0 to 7.5. It is easy to grow from seed, either direct-sown or started indoors. You can also propagate it by making root divisions of established plants. To prevent self-sowing, deadhead the plants after bloom. *Zones 3–8.*

Harvesting. Harvest the roots from established colonies in autumn, or at any other time when the plants are not in bloom. Fresh use is preferred, but soapwort roots can be grated and dried.

SOUTHERNWOOD *Artemisia abrotanum*

Also known as: Old man, lad's love, maid's ruin, lover's plant, *garderobe*

Plant type: Perennial

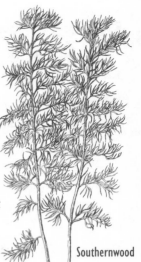
Southernwood

In the language of flowers, southernwood stands for affectionate fidelity, a love that withstands the test of time and trials. In the Middle Ages, it was one of the popular strewing herbs, repelling insects and providing fragrance and soft footing in both castles and cottages. It was also considered an aphrodisiac, and so was brewed into love potions and included in bouquets sent to lovers. A hundred years ago a young man going courting often wore a sprig in his hat to announce his intentions. Southernwood has an unusual fragrance, blending a little lemon with a lot of camphor.

Uses. Southernwood is an insect repellent, so hang branches in pantries and closets or lay it along shelves. Also, lay dry branches under wool rugs, and use it in sachets, wreaths, garlands, and tussie-mussies. Dry it carefully to add to everlasting arrangements. Use it fresh or dried in water, vinegar, ammonia, or alcohol extractions.

In the garden. Southernwood is a sprawling, multistemmed perennial shrub, 3 to 5 feet tall, with a 2- to 3-foot spread. It has very fine, feathery, gray-green foliage. It rarely blooms in northern gardens; in the South it has yellowish flowers. Southernwood needs well-drained soil with a pH of 5.5 to 7.5, and full sun. Space plants about 3 feet apart, and control their sprawl by tying them back or pruning. Southernwood rarely sets seed, and when it does, viability is poor, so propagate by root division in the spring or fall, or propagate young plants by layering. Southernwood keeps its silver color throughout the seasons, a lovely contrast to spring greens and bronze hues of autumn. If you'd like a hedge of southernwood, space plants 2 feet apart. *Zones 4–9.*

Harvesting. Harvest by cutting 1- or 2-foot stems early in the season, and take another cutting later. Prune straggling branches near the base. Hang-dry in bundles or lay them flat on a rack to dry.

SPEARMINT *Mentha spicata*

Also known as: Garden mint, lamb mint, spire mint, green mint
Plant type: Perennial

This mint lacks the biting pungency of peppermint because it contains no menthol. It is therefore the safest mint for pregnant women and small children.

Uses. Spearmint is antibacterial, antiviral, and antiparasitical, although it is somewhat weaker than peppermint. Use fresh or dried spearmint in water, vinegar, ammonia, and alcohol extractions for surface cleaning. It can also be used in potpourris.

Spearmint

In the garden. A hardy perennial herb, spearmint grows to 3 feet. It has the square stem typical of all the mints, oval green leaves, and a spire of pale mauve flowers. Set plants a foot apart in full sun to partial shade in moist soil, pH 7.0 to 8.0. Mulch to keep the soil moist and promote the creation of runners. Use only composted manure, since fresh manure encourages rust. To grow spearmint indoors, pot the plants but then leave them outside in the cold for at least a 2-month dormant period before bringing them inside. *Zones 3–9.*

Harvesting. Harvest established mint freely, cutting back one third to half of the plant early in the year to encourage branching. Clip again when in bloom, and harvest entire stems that have gotten out of bounds. Bundle and hang-dry, or dry sprigs on a rack.

SWEET ANNIE *Artemisia annua*

Also known as: Christmas tree herb
Plant type: Annual

If you let it go to seed, sweet Annie may spread all over your garden. I've had it grow among the patio bricks, between the cracks of the sidewalk, and into the thyme bed. But it's a crafter's favorite, with a delightful fragrance — light, sweet, and penetrating. The fragrance holds whether harvested or left to age in the garden.

Sweet Annie

Uses. An effective antiseptic, sweet Annie kills common fungi and yeasts that cause skin infections, and a parasitic bacteria *(Leptospira)* that affects humans, dogs, pigs, horses, and cattle. It contains an acid that acts against staph, salmonella, *E. coli*, and other bacteria. Use the diluted essential oil to disinfect surfaces. The Chinese burn the dried herb to kill mosquitoes. In the West, sweet Annie is often used for crafts, including tussie-mussies, wreath bases, and herbal candles. I like to use it in simmering potpourri with sacred basil (another reputed mosquito chaser), chamomile, linden, and orange peel.

In the garden. Full-grown annual sweet Annie can be as tall as 6 feet and as wide as 3 feet at the base. It has lacy leaves, with fernlike divisions. Start seed indoors or directly in the garden, or buy a plant or two. Let plants go to seed and they'll produce plenty of extras for harvesting. Sweet Annie thrives in just about any soil with average drainage in full sun. Plants crowded together (1 foot apart) produce more disinfecting compounds, but if you want to make wreaths, give them a 3-foot spacing so the foliage has room to develop fully.

Harvesting. Harvest leaves any time after midsummer, by either collecting the lower leaves or lopping off the tops of the plants. They'll branch out and regrow to provide you with another harvest. Collect plants for disinfectant applications just as the flowers start to bud, because the antimalarial compound artemisinin in sweet Annie is at its highest level at this time. Harvest the entire plant before the first frost. Use fresh or hang-dry bundles in the dark for ornamental uses, since exposure to light darkens the plant considerably.

SWEET GRASS *Hierochloe odorata,* *H. odorata fragrans*

Also known as: Seneca grass, holy grass, vanilla grass, Indian hay
Plant type: Hardy perennial

Sweet Grass

Sweet grass has a delicious fragrance. When fresh, it smells like new-mown hay, but drying intensifies the scent and brings out a vanilla aroma.
Uses. Native Americans use sweet grass to make storage baskets, boxes, and mats, and they burn it in ceremonies to purify the atmosphere. Place braids in dresser drawers, chests, or closets to repel insects. Sweet grass is a fixative: try it in potpourris and sachets. Dried sweet grass is better than fresh for making water, vinegar, ammonia, and alcohol extractions. I especially like the extra fruity scent and deep, orange-red color it develops when extracted in vinegar for use as an air freshener (see Vinegar Bowl, page 123).
In the garden. This cold-hardy plant needs rich, moist soil, high in nitrogen: its native conditions are wet prairies and meadows. A beautiful hardy perennial, sweet grass sports long, narrow green leaves with a definite midrib. It grows to 2 or 3 feet tall, and spreads rapidly underground. Nurseries specializing in native plants sell 3-inch plugs, which can spread 1 to 2 feet in diameter in their first growing season. You can separate the individual rhizomes in the plugs for wider coverage. Weed vigilantly. *Zones 4–9.*
Harvesting. Harvest by shearing off the grass blades with scissors, then dry them flat on a rack, or rubber-band the stems tightly and hang to dry. If you're planning to braid the grass, keep the cut ends pointed in the same direction, hang-dry them, then soak them in water for about an hour to make them more pliable.

Sweet Woodruff *Galium odoratum*

Also known as: Woodrove, *Waldmeister* (master of the woods), herb Walter, hay plant, star grass, *muguet de bois* (musk of the woods)

Plant type: Hardy perennial

Sweet woodruff's leaf whorls inspired many of the plant's common names. The plant was called woodruff because its whorls reminded Elizabethans of the stiff lace ruffs so popular with the upper classes. The "rove" in woodrove derives from a French word, *rovelle,* meaning "wheel"; to the French, sweet woodruff's leaves looked like the spokes in a wagon wheel.

Sweet Woodruff

Sweet woodruff's fragrance is a beautiful blend of vanilla and fresh-cut hay, but the scent is almost undetectable in the fresh leaves unless they are crushed. The scent develops fully only when the leaves are cut and the drying process begins.

Uses. Add to potpourri, perfumes, and sachet blends as a fixative. As a decorative herb, use it in wreaths and garlands. For its aroma, stuff sweet woodruff into sleep pillows and use in sweet bags (see pages 130–31). Lay sprigs on pantry, closet, and book shelves, and spread under wool rugs to deter insects; and use it fresh or dried in water, vinegar, ammonia, or alcohol extractions for air fresheners.

In the garden. A short, hardy perennial ground cover, usually about 6 to 9 inches tall, sweet woodruff is a natural traveler, spreading by surface runners and shallow underground roots. Tiny, fragrant, waxy white flowers bloom in May or early June. Sweet woodruff will grow in a mass in a moist, shady, humus-rich location with a pH of 5.0. By nature a woodland plant, sweet woodruff thrives in dappled sunlight. Side-dress plants with composted leaves. *Zones 3–9.*

Harvesting. Harvest flowering sprigs for May wine in spring. Gather the tops of several plants in one hand and use scissors to shear them off, leaving at least two whorls of leaves below, so that the plants can recover and branch out. Later in the summer, harvest again. Sweet woodruff is usually used after drying. I spread it in a shallow basket right in my living room, turning the plants daily, so that it perfumes the air for all to enjoy as it dries. Store in glass jars until needed.

TANSY *Tanacetum vulgare*
Also known as: Bitter buttons, ant fern
Plant type: Perennial

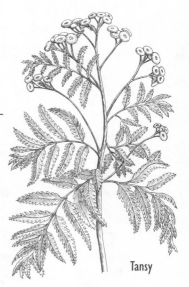

Tansy

Tansy leaves are pungent, rather than fragrant. In early Scotland, tansy was incorporated into granaries to keep mice out. It is also said to deter flies, fleas, and ants. Because the essential oil contains a high percentage of thujone and camphor, the oil should not be used for housekeeping tasks. On the other hand, the dried leaves are excellent insect chasers.

Uses. Tansy extracts repel beetles, according to tests done at Lehigh University, so it's a good companion plant in an organic garden. Extract it in water, vinegar, ammonia, or alcohol. It may also act as a good surface wash to control pinworms and roundworms. Collect the flowers when newly opened for wreaths and arrangements.

In the garden. This perennial herb grows 4 feet tall and about 2 or 3 feet wide. Tansy has numerous floppy stems covered in dark-green, fernlike leaves. It blooms in August and September with flat, egg-yolk-yellow buttons without petals. It grows in almost any soil with a pH of 5.0 to 7.5 in full sun. It's easiest to grow from root divisions, but you can also grow it from seed or cuttings. Its rhizomes spread aggressively, and once it's established, it's hard to get rid of it. Plant it where it has plenty of room, or provide boundaries, such as underground pots, to keep its roots from spreading, so that it doesn't ruin your garden design. *Zones 3–9.*

Harvesting. Harvest leaves as plants go into bud, and use it fresh or dried. Hang to dry.

THYME *Thymus vulgaris*

Also known as: Common thyme
Plant type: Perennial

One of the most familiar and popular culinary herbs, thyme is also a dependable garden plant, especially when featured as a ground cover or allowed to creep over stone walls or in container plantings.

Uses. Because thyme's essential oil contains a crystalline component called thymol, it has strong disinfectant and antibacterial properties. It also acts against some fungi, the virus that causes shingles, and intestinal parasites like roundworms and hookworms. Studies now show that it is also effective on mosquito larvae. Use fresh or dried leaves in water, vinegar, ammonia, and alcohol extractions to clean and disinfect. Shrubby bunches of thyme make good culinary wreath bases and garlands. Lemon thyme *(Thymus × citriodorus)* — my favorite for housekeeping — is very expensive and not always commercially available, so it really pays to grow your own.

In the garden. A small, shrubby, upright perennial, thyme has many woody stems. It grows to 1 foot high with a similar spread. Leaves are small (¼ to ½ inch long), shiny, dark green, and strongly scented. Small pinkish lilac to purple flowers blossom in June and July. Propagate from seed, cuttings, layering, or root divisions taken in spring only. Thyme likes a light, sandy, well-drained soil with a pH of 6.0 to 8.0, and prefers full sun, although it will tolerate very lightly dappled shade. Mulch plants, and cover them to protect from frost heaving and winter winds. Once plants are established, clip them frequently to encourage new growth and to prevent woody stems. Thymes are short-lived and may need to be replaced every few years. *Zones 2–9.*

Harvesting. University studies have established that the essential oil is most potent in plant material harvested in July and August, which are good times to shear back the plants. Leave a few inches, and then water to encourage new growth. If you take a second cutting (chancy even from well-established plants), be sure to provide plenty of winter protection.

WINTER SAVORY *Satureja montana*
Also known as: Bean herb
Plant type: Perennial

In addition to its household uses, winter savory attracts pollinators to your garden — bees love it. It repels parasites and has antibacterial properties.

Uses. Use the fresh or dried stems in water, vinegar, ammonia, and alcohol extractions for surface cleaning. Winter savory is also a useful everlasting, makes a good culinary wreath base, and can be incorporated into garlands.

Winter Savory

In the garden. This small, shrubby perennial herb is slow-growing, semi-evergreen, and upright. It grows a little over 1 foot high and wide, with a tendency to sprawl when it's older. The aromatic leaves are shiny and dark green. It bears white flowers from July through early September. Start from seed indoors eight weeks before the soil warms, or take cuttings or root divisions from established plants in the spring; space plants about 1 foot apart. Savory requires full sun and well-drained soil with a pH of 6.7 to 7.0. Winter savory makes a nice edging for garden beds. Care for it as described for thyme. *Zones 4–9.*

If you want savory in your garden, but don't have an established winter savory plant, you can grow summer savory, the taller annual species, *S. hortensis.* It requires the same conditions as *S. montana.*

Harvesting. Treat winter savory as described for thyme, taking up to two clippings of established plants per year. You can clip annual summer savory several times, and the entire plant can be harvested at the end of the summer, but allow at least one to bloom and set seed for next year's garden.

WORMWOOD *Artemisia absinthium*

Also known as: Absinthe, green ginger
Plant type: Perennial shrub

This herb has a somewhat mixed reputation. When used to flavor an alcoholic, mood-altering drink called absinthe, its toxic properties can cause convulsions and even death. U.S. law prohibited the sale of absinthe in 1912. Toulouse-Lautrec depicted its effects in his Parisian café paintings, in which he shows green-skinned, cadaverous people drinking the addictive nar-cotic. But wormwood also has benefits: its antiseptic and insect-chasing powers make it useful in surface-cleaning solutions and protective sachets. It has a distinctive, aromatic fragrance.

Wormwood

Uses. Powdered wormwood seed repels fleas and protects books from parasites. The dried leaves repel wool moths and deter the hatching of their larvae. Hang branches of the plant in pantries and closets, or lay them along bookshelves. Extract it in water, vinegar, ammonia, or alcohol. Wormwood is a useful antiseptic for surface cleaning. It can also be used in wreaths and sachets.

Safety first. Never ingest any solution containing wormwood. If you are pregnant, avoid using wormwood extractions. Do not use it on surfaces small children touch.

In the garden. Wormwood, a greenish gray perennial shrub, grows in clumps to a height of 4 feet with a spread of about 2 feet. In August or September, its tiny yellow blossoms contrast with its silvery leaves. In late fall or winter, it dies back to the root. Wormwood appreciates a loamy soil with some clay in it and will grow just about anywhere with a pH of 5.5 to 7.5 in full sun. It will even tolerate some dappled shade. It doesn't set much viable seed, so propagate by root division of an established plant in spring or fall, take cuttings from new growth in March or October, or buy a plant from a reputable supplier. Plant it 1 foot away from other plants in all directions, as the absinthin com-pound in its leaves will inhibit the growth of nearby plants. *Zones 4–9.*

Harvesting. Harvest wormwood branches for drying in late summer, as it comes into bud. Cut snippets to be used fresh in water, vinegar, or alcohol extractions any time.

YARROW *Achillea millefolium*

Also known as: Achillea, milfoil, woundwort, yarroway, carpenter's weed, knight's milfoil, soldier's woundwort, old man's pepper, sneezewort

Plant type: Hardy perennial

In the Scottish Hebrides, yarrow was used in charms to foretell the future, and was also commonly used in sleep pillows to give visions of the true love's face. The Saxons sewed it into amulets to use as a charm against all misfortunes. As a companion plant, yarrow enhances the essential oil production of other herbs that grow nearby.

Yarrow

Uses. Yarrow tea is often used to water ailing plants. Mildly disinfectant and astringent, it's used in water, vinegar, ammonia, or alcohol extractions for surface cleaning. The essential oil tends to be too expensive for most household uses, but it makes a good insect chaser for moths, roaches, or mosquitoes.

In the garden. Yarrow is a hardy perennial with erect rough stems covered with fine, silky hairs. It has fernlike grayish green leaves, 3 to 4 inches long and about 1 inch wide, and bears numerous tiny white (or occasionally pinkish) daisylike blossoms, crowded together in a flat flowerhead, from June to September. Yarrow tends to self-sow, and some gardeners find it invasive. Yarrow grows easily from seed (which requires light to germinate) and from root divisions, which you can make in early spring or autumn. Plant in full sun, in average, well-drained soil (it will tolerate poor soil) with a pH of 4.2 to 7.0, spacing plants about a foot or less apart. *Zones 3–10.*

Harvesting. Although the whole plant can be used, I tend to use the leaves and flowering stalks, harvested as needed throughout the summer. Process fresh, or hang-dry stems for later use.

YUCCA *Yucca glauca*

Also known as: Soapweed, soapwell
Plant type: Hardy perennial

Yucca's dramatic flowers are especially fragrant at night. The leaves can be split and used to make baskets. Its root, rich in soapy saponins, was featured in a Native American wedding ceremony ritual during which the bride and groom shampooed each other's hair. A delightfully sensual tradition!

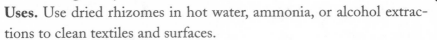

Yucca

Uses. Use dried rhizomes in hot water, ammonia, or alcohol extractions to clean textiles and surfaces.

In the garden. A hardy evergreen perennial, yucca grows from a thick underground rhizome. Its 16- to 28-inch-long, stiff, pointed leaves radiate from a basal rosette. From May to July, the 2- to 3-inch, creamy or greenish white, bell-like flowers are borne on a long stalk that rises well above the leaves. Propagate yucca by sowing fresh, ripe seed or from side shoots, stem cuttings, rhizomes, or root divisions taken in spring. Plant yucca in full sun, in light, sandy loam with good drainage, and space in clumps every 3 or 4 feet. Becuase yucca can get along with very little water, it's an excellent plant for dry climates. *Zones 4–10.*

Harvesting. Harvest the rhizomes from plants large enough to set side shoots in the early spring, and replant the shoots. For best rhizome production, cut flower buds off the plants so they can't set seed. Clean, peel, grate, and dry the rhizome. Powdered root is available from health food stores and suppliers.

TREES AND SHRUBS WITH HERBAL USES

In addition to the herbs described in the preceding pages, the leaves, barks, seeds, and roots of a number of common trees and shrubs also have characteristics that make them helpful household herbs. Refer to the chart that follows for some of the most popular, which you may already have growing on your property.

Herbal Uses of Some Trees and Shrubs at a Glance

HERB	PART USED	USES
Blue gum eucalyptus (*Eucalyptus globulus*)	Leaves	Insect chaser, potpourri and simmering potpourri, surface wash; essential oil is intensely antibiotic, antiviral, antifungal
European elder (*Sambucus nigra*)	Flowers, leaves, bark	Potpourri and simmering potpourri, surface wash
Fir (*Abies* species)	Needles	Fumigant, incense, simmering potpourri
Frankincense (*Boswellia carterii*)	Gum	Fumigant, incense, potpourri and simmering potpourri
Ginkgo (*Ginkgo biloba*)	Leaves	Insect chaser, surface wash
Juniper (*Juniperus communis*)	Needles	Incense, potpourri and simmering potpourri, surface wash
Linden (*Tilia x europaea*)	Flowers, bracts	Potpourri and simmering potpourri, surface wash
Myrrh (*Commiphora myrrha*)	Resin	Fumigant, incense, potpourri
Neem (*Azadirachta indica*)	Leaves	Agricultural uses; plant drench, surface wash
Pine (*Pinus* species)	Needles	Fumigant, incense, simmering potpourri
Prickly ash (*Zanthoxylum americanum*)	Bark, berries	Insect chaser, surface wash
Red cedar (*Juniperus virginiana*)	Needles, wood	Fumigant, incense, insect chaser, potpourri and simmering potpourri
Sandalwood (*Santalum album*)	Wood	Insect chaser, potpourri and simmering potpourri, surface wash
Spruce (*Picea* species)	Needles	Fumigant, incense, simmering potpourri
Witch hazel (*Hamamelis virginiana*)	Bark, twigs, leaves	Surface wash

Where to Find Housekeeping Recipes

TYPE	RECIPES	PAGE
Air fresheners	Deodorizers	123–24
	Potpourris	132–33
	Sprays	125–26
Bathroom and kitchen cleaners	Disinfectants	126
	Scouring powders	91–93
	Surface cleaners	93–95
Carpet and rug care	Fresheners	100–1
	Insect pest controls	102–3
Glass treatment	Scratch remover	98
	Cleaners	97
Laundry aids	Laundry powders	118–19
	Presoaks	118
	Soaps	95–96, 109–10
Leather care	Cleaners	120–21
	Conditioners	121–23
Metal polishes	Various	99–100
Pest control	Deterrents	128–31
	Treatments	102–3
Scented crafts	Various	127–34
Stain treatments	Stain removers	113–17
	Stain pretreatments	115–17
Floor and furniture care	Cleaners and polishes	103–7
	Waxes	107–9

CHAPTER 4

GROWING HERBS
for Natural Cleaning

Growing your own herbs is rewarding in so many ways. When I walk through my garden, I feel a real sense of pride and accomplishment. Being outside and surrounded by aromatic herbs, I feel soothed and connected to nature through the colors, textures, scents, and shapes of the plants I love. A delightful extension of my home, my garden provides many materials to beautify and clean in a way that supports my family's health.

I've created four herb garden designs to provide you with different options that you can use or adapt to suit your own needs, interests, and available space. These designs, combined with advice on how to grow your herbs from seed to harvest, should pave the way to your own success with herbs.

STARTING HERBS FROM SEED

Whether you start seeds indoors to get a head start on the season, or sow them directly in the garden beds where they will grow, you'll save money by growing your own plants from scratch rather than buying young herbs at a nursery. You will probably also have a greater variety of herbs to choose from.

DIRECT-SEEDING ANNUALS

Borage, caraway (biennial), chervil (do not cover with soil; it requires light to germinate), coriander, cumin, epazoté, fenugreek, nigella, perilla, and sweet Annie all flourish when planted in the garden where they will grow. Anise, dill, and fennel, which have long taproots and tender stems, resent transplanting, and must be direct-seeded.

Planting bed. If the soil in your herb bed is too acidic, add ground limestone; if it's too alkaline, add powdered sulfur or ammonium sulfate. Follow package directions for the amount to use. These are only temporary remedies. For long-term soil health, add compost annually. If your soil lacks humus, add compost or composted manure. Heavy clay soils are unsuitable for herb gardens; the best way to counter this situation is to build raised beds and fill them with a combination of good topsoil and compost, which will provide better drainage.

Sowing method. After the soil has warmed and all danger of frost has passed, prepare the soil in your herb bed. Seeds germinate most reliably in fine-textured soil, dug to a depth of about a foot, then raked and sifted to remove stones and debris. Press seeds gently into the soil, then barely cover them with finely sifted soil or a thin layer of clean sand, no deeper than the seed's own diameter. Water carefully with a fine mist. For the first watering, use hot water to promote germination. Don't allow the bed to dry out. After they germinate, thin seedlings to the spacing described for each plant in Chapter 3, beginning on page 27.

Cover newly sown seeds with sand.

DIRECT-SEEDING PERENNIALS

Many perennials also do well from seed. The usual method is to plant seeds outdoors (in a cold frame if possible), or in a prepared, protected seedbed. Consider direct-sowing anise hyssop, bee balm, betony, catnip, chives, comfrey, coneflower (first stratify seed; see box below), dianthus, elecampane, horehound, hyssop, lemon balm, lovage, mugwort, nepeta, oregano, rue, sage, salad burnet, soapwort, sorrel, tansy, thyme, valerian, winter savory, wormwood, and yarrow. Biennial angelica is also easily grown from stratified seed.

Sowing method. Sow seed in late spring or early summer, so young plants can grow and harden off for a few months before going dormant for the winter. When seedlings have at least two sets of true leaves, thin them, and pinch back buds to encourage leaf growth and root development. Make sure they have enough water, wind protection, and fertilizer to become well established. Don't fertilize toward the end of the growing season; tender new growth will not be able to withstand the stresses of winter. In early autumn, transplant the young plants to their permanent growing site. They will bloom for the first time the following year.

Stratifying Seed

Some seeds need to undergo a period of chilling before they'll germinate (see advice about specific herbs in Chapter 3, starting on page 27). To simulate winter, put seeds in a small, covered glass jar in the freezer for 1 to 2 months before planting.

STARTING TENDER ANNUALS AND PERENNIALS INDOORS

Not all young herbs can withstand the rigors of cold temperatures and drying winds. Start delicate annuals, such as chamomile, basil, calendula, marigold, nasturtium, epazoté, and summer savory, indoors under grow lights. Even taprooted annuals like anise can be started indoors if your climate is extremely cold, with a short growing season.

You'll need to sow such seeds directly into 4-inch or deeper pots, and when you transplant them to the garden, use a wind and sun shelter, such as a cloche, row cover fabric (such as Reemay), or even a strategically placed piece of cardboard stapled to sticks pounded into the earth, while the plant establishes itself. You can also give an indoor start to all the hardy perennials mentioned on page 65 under Direct-Seeding Perennials, usually in January or February. Be prepared, however, to provide them with high light levels and months of attention.

Timing. Sow seed indoors about six to eight weeks before the last frost date for your region. In my Zone 5, that means no later than about mid-March. It's important not to sow too early, or herbs will outgrow their pots and become rootbound before it's time to transplant them.

Planting mixture. To sow plants indoors, purchase soilless seed-starting mix, or blend your own. The mixture must be light, fine textured, and porous, as many herb seeds are very small. Pro-Mix is a popular commercial product. Or make your own mix, typically of

Money-Saving Lights

An inexpensive indoor rig for growing and starting seeds doesn't require fancy lightbulbs. You can create an almost equivalent balance of light wavelengths by putting one warm and one cool bulb (usually 40-watt) in a fluorescent shop light. Set up the lights on an adjustable chain. If the seeds need light to germinate, hang the lights about 3 inches from the top of the flat before germination; when seedlings appear, keep adjusting the lights so they're always 3 inches above the plant leaves.

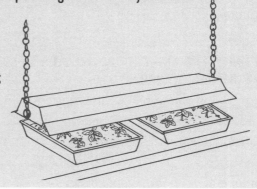

equal parts milled peat moss, vermiculite, and perlite. (Blend small amounts in a dishpan or 5-gallon bucket. For larger amounts, use a shovel and mix in a wheelbarrow.) This soilless mix is sterile, which means it contains no disease organisms to promote damping-off of seedlings or root rot. However, it also contains no nutrients, so it's not suitable as a potting mix for older plants unless you intend to feed them frequently with liquid fertilizer.

Containers. Collect recycled ½- to ¾-inch-deep containers for seed trays, or purchase seed-starting trays if you are starting a large number of seeds at one time. Make drainage slits in the bottom of each tray. Sterilize all containers in a 5% solution of household bleach.

Labels. Because you're likely to have wet, dirty hands once you get into the sowing process, make up labels for each type of seed you are planting before you open any seed packets. I use an indelible marker on Popsicle sticks, but recycled plastic from milk cartons or soft drink bottles works well, too.

Sorting seeds. It's also helpful to sort seeds according to whether they require covering, so you can keep together all seeds with the same light requirements. For best results, follow the directions on your seed packets or in the individual plant descriptions in Chapter 3, starting on page 27.

Providing warmth. I always presoak seed in warm water (at or slightly above body temperature, no hotter). Think of this step as imitating a warm spring rainfall. Put the seed in labeled paper cups or small baby-food jars, pour the warm water over the seeds, and let them stand overnight. The next day, pour out most of the water through a fine tea strainer, leaving the seeds in a small bit of water in the bottom of the container. Dump the seeds and remaining water into a bowl, so you can use tweezers or your thumb and index finger to pick up the tiny seeds.

Pick up small seeds from presoak water with tweezers.

Moisten seed-starting mix with very hot, even boiling, water. Use a wooden paint stirrer or other tool to mix thoroughly. It should be moist but not sopping. Allow to cool to lukewarm before sowing seeds.

I also use root-zone heater cables (available from garden suppliers) to keep the bottom of the seedling flat at 75°–80°F; if you don't have cables, the top of the refrigerator will provide some extra warmth. This, combined with a warm presoak and a warm planting medium, often provides germination in as little as two to three days. Notorious slow-starters like parsley take seven to ten days.

Sowing method. Fill the seed flats so that the soilless mix is about 2 inches deep. Press down the mixture lightly to remove any large air holes. Gently thump smaller flats against the work surface and shake them from side to side to settle the mixture. Then smooth the surface, using your fingers to gently press down the soil.

Sow seed on the surface, using your thumb and index finger to scatter the seeds. If you have trouble spacing small seeds, place them in a teaspoon and, holding it just over the flat, use the tip of a sharpened pencil or tweezers to nudge the seeds off the spoon. Mix really tiny seeds with a tablespoon of sterile sand before sowing.

Sow small seed from a teaspoon.

Try to space seeds at least ½ inch or more apart; it will make transplanting much easier if their roots aren't entangled. Use the palm or edge of your hand to press the seeds gently into the planting mix. Cover larger seeds with a fine layer of milled peat moss or sterile sand.

Press seed into planting mix.

Seedling care. Water with a fine mist, using the seedling rose on your watering can or a spray bottle. Cover the flat with glass or plastic wrap to retain moisture. Remove the covering once seedlings have germinated. If you have sown different types of plants in the same flat, it's unlikely that they will all germinate or be ready for transplanting at the same time. You may have to cover half or a quarter of the flat and leave the rest open. After seeds germinate, continue to water trays as needed. Bottom watering is best at this point, but if that's not possible, use a seedling rose to provide a fine mist.

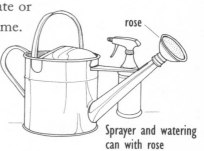

rose

Sprayer and watering can with rose

Recent research suggests that seedlings will be healthiest if provided with half-strength liquid fertilizer, such as manure tea, kelp, or fish emulsion, once a week. Good air circulation is also crucial to growing healthy plants. Set a household fan to move air around the area, but don't let it blow directly on young plants.

Transplanting. Two to four weeks after seedlings germinate, they form their first set of true leaves. Once this happens, transplant the young seedlings to larger pots filled with a potting soil mix. The soil blend for transplants does not need to be sterile or soilless; at this stage, plants are less susceptible to damping-off. The usual mix is equal parts loam, sieved compost, and perlite or vermiculite. (Research shows that sieved compost battles fungi that promote damping-off disease and also provides nitrogen to tender seedlings. Don't use more than one-third compost, however, as it tends to have a high level of salt.)

Prevent Damping-Off

Newly germinated seedlings or young plants that suddenly fall over are victims of damping-off, which is caused by microorganisms. Remove dead plants from the flat immediately to keep the condition from spreading. Prevent damping-off by using sterilized planting media and equipment. Misting seedlings with strong chamomile tea may also be helpful.

Before transplanting tiny seedlings, allow the soil to dry out slightly so that it's easier to remove the tender roots without damaging them. Fill pots with soil mix and use your finger to poke a hole big enough to insert the tiny plant. Always grasp the seedling by its top set of true leaves, rather than the stem. If the leaves break off, the buds on the stem will sprout, thus saving the plant; if the stem breaks below the first set of true leaves, however, the plant will die.

Hold plant by top leaves during trans-planting.

Gently shake the seed-starting mix off the roots and lower the roots into the prepared hole. Firm the soil mix around the roots, adding more soil if necessary. Water well and replace under lights.

Care of transplants. New transplants aren't too demanding. Water them in the morning, then keep them under lights for 12 to 14 hours a day. As they mature, you may direct a house-hold fan near or on them. Feed them every week with a diluted water-soluble organic fertilizer.

Pinching back encourages bushiness. Once the plant has three sets of true leaves, pinch off the top set to force side-shoot production. Then pinch back side shoots when they have two sets of leaves. Continue pinching back all plants as they need it.

Pinch back to encourage bushiness.

MOVING OUTDOORS

Whether you have started seed indoors or purchased greenhouse-grown plants, once the outdoor soil is warm and temperatures have moderated, it's time to move seedling plants outside. To harden off plants for a week before transplanting, place them in a spot that gets limited sunlight and is protected from wind. Gradually expose them to more of the elements by leaving them out longer in less and less sheltered spots each day. This process strengthens the delicate "skins" of plants that have been grown indoors, actually thickening their cells so they can withstand the elements.

Plants with Special Soil-Mix Needs

- Substitute milled peat moss for perlite when growing woodland shade plants, such as sweet woodruff, which prefer an acidic soil.
- Add sand and coarsely ground limestone (screenings) to the mix for plants like thyme, lavender, and horehound, which require limy, gritty, well-drained soil. If you use soil blocks rather than plastic or clay pots, follow this ratio: 1 part builder's sand, 1 part compost, and 2 parts soil. Peat moss is not included in these mixes, so that water will percolate through them quickly. Most herbs (calamus is an exception) can't tolerate water standing around their roots.

Planting day. Pinch off any flower buds. When plants are newly set, their energy should be directed toward establishing roots, not flowers. Dig planting holes of the right size and spacing before unpotting your transplants. A rule of thumb is to place tall, thin plants so that the distance between full-grown plants will be half their height. Short, wide plants should be spaced so that the distance between plants will be twice their mature height, which will give them room to spread. Site plants according to the information in the individual plant profiles in Chapter 3. Sometimes commercially grown plants are rootbound from being left in their pots too long. Shake off the growing mix, then untangle the roots and spread them out carefully.

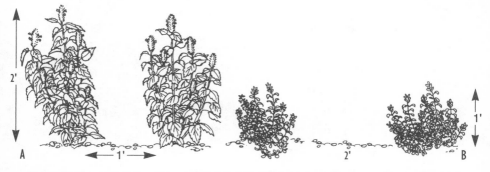

Place tall mints at half the distance of their height (A); place short thymes at twice the distance of their height (B).

LONG-TERM CARE

Once your transplants are in place, keep them well watered so they don't dry out. Also, protect them from wind until they are established. Continue to shape perennial plants by pinching them back throughout the growing season. I never allow any first-year perennials to bloom. Pinching off all buds forces perennial plants to establish strong root systems and a lot of upper growth.

Watering. Once plants are established, I rely on natural rainfall and a mulch to keep the ground moist between rains. This forces plants to send their roots deep into the soil, keeping them healthier and more drought-resistant than if their feeder roots stayed near the surface, reliant upon top watering. I make an exception and use a soaker hose on roses if we have a dry period while they're in bloom.

Weeding. Weed carefully around young plants to reduce competition. When the soil has warmed sufficiently, apply a 4-inch layer of mulch. (Leave a couple of inches of space around the base of each plant so that collected moisture doesn't cause plants to rot.)

Fertilizing. My garden needs little extra fertilizer, although I sometimes sprinkle powdered kelp around plants just before a rain. How often you fertilize will depend on your soil conditions. Place compost or composted manure over a newly established bed, then add some once again each year thereafter.

Preparing for winter. In early winter, after the ground freezes, I pile straw or leaves deeply on dormant plants like roses and lavenders that require protection from winter winds and frost heaves. Like most northern farmers, I love to see a nice, thick, reliable coat of snow on the ground, but we don't always get what we want, so the straw is insurance against drying winds and freeze-thaw cycles.

Mulch sage with straw for winter protection.

GARDENING IN CONTAINERS

If you garden on a patio or balcony, you will have to transplant overgrown plants to larger containers. Select pots big enough to hold the plants and allow for more growth, usually about 2 inches larger than the original pot. Since herbs require really good drainage, I use rather tall clay pots, ranging in depth from 6 to 15 inches, depending on the size of the plant, and put 2 inches of limestone screenings or tailings (available at building supply stores) in the bottom of each pot.

Fill pots about one-half to two-thirds full of soil mix. Mound some soil (like a tiny mountain) in the center of the pot. Carefully spread the plant's roots over the mound, then fill the pot with soil, press it down gently but firmly, and thump the pot a few times to settle the soil around the roots. Water thoroughly.

When you bring established container plants indoors for the winter, it may help to prune both the tops and roots. To do this, first cut the top back severely by half or more. Then, remove the plant from its pot and trim back its roots by about one-third. Repot the plant in new soil. Use the trimmings in sachets, potpourris, or other projects, or to make extractions to use in cleaning formulas.

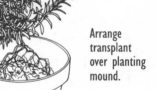

Magnificent Mints

Mints benefit from being left out in the cold for two months of dormancy before being brought inside.

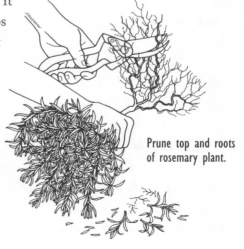

Arrange transplant over planting mound.

Prune top and roots of rosemary plant.

LANDSCAPING WITH HOUSEKEEPING HERBS

Herb gardens meant for utilitarian purposes can be beautiful elements of any residential landscape. The four gardens shown here vary in size from a grouping of container plants for a deck or patio to a large, L-shaped shrub border, but all the designs can be modified to fit the space you have available.

Site. Since most herbs are sun lovers, it's important to site your garden with its long axis running north–south in an area that gets 8 to 10 hours or more of sun daily. Note how trees, fences, buildings, and other structures that shade the garden. In the north, the south side of a building is usually a wonderful place to establish an herb garden. The building both provides protection from winter winds and radiates additional warmth to plants. What works like a charm in Illinois, however, may be a disaster in hot, dry southern Arizona or hot, humid Florida, so check with the local chapter of the Herb Society of America or your county Cooperative Extension Service for advice on growing an herb garden in your region. For information about individual plants in these designs, consult Chapter 3, Housekeeping Herbs A to Z, starting on page 27.

FRUIT-SCENTED CONTAINER GARDEN

A fruit-scented garden can be a prized and very enjoyable feature of any south-, east-, or even west-facing balcony, patio, courtyard, deck, or porch. To make more plant material available, grow masses of a single kind of plant in a large pot. Remember that the mints and scented geraniums will appreciate dappled sunlight.

Maintenance. Plant mints and chamomile in large pots and pinch them back frequently to encourage branching. Keep lemon basils pinched back so they don't bloom. The tropical sages, scented geraniums, and basils are all tender perennials, and if kept long enough they will develop woody stems. Pinch them back frequently to shape them nicely before they mature.

Winter care. In areas where temperatures fall below 40°F, all these plants will have to be brought in for the winter and kept under grow lights. Trim back the tops by at least half, then unpot the plant and trim back a third of the roots. Repot in new soil before moving indoors. Leave the mints outside for the required two-month dormancy before bringing them in. Repot them in new soil before taking them outside again. The lemon tree needs well-drained soil, so use a light potting soil containing perlite and compost or peat moss. Indoors, place it where it gets sunlight at least half the day, and temperatures between 40–75°F.

Fruit-Scented Container Garden

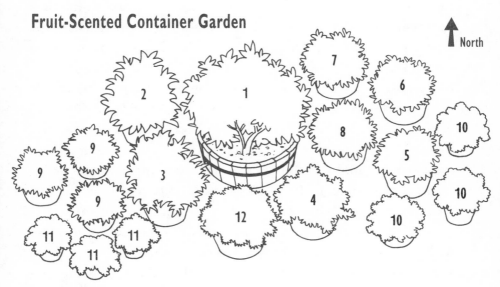

1. Lemon tree (*Citrus limon*), 1*
2. Fruit-scented sage (*Salvia dorisiana*), 1
3. Pineapple sage (*Salvia elegans*), 1
4. Lemon balm (*Melissa officinalis*), 1
5. Applemint (*Mentha suaveolens*), 6–12
6. Orangemint (*Mentha x piperita* 'Citrata'), 6–12
7. Pineapple mint (*Mentha suaveolens* 'Variegata'), 6–12
8. Lemon mint (*Mentha x aquatica* 'Citrata'), 6–12
9. Lemon basil (*Ocimum basilicum* var. *citriodorum*), 3–6
10. Lemon geranium (*Pelargonium radens*), 3–6
11. Lemon thyme (*Thymus citriodorus*), 3–6
12. Chamomile (*Matricaria recutita*), 6–12

OPTIONAL:
Orange tree (*Citrus sinensis*), 1
Lemon verbena (*Aloysia triphylla*), 1
Orange balsam thyme (*Thymus vulgaris* 'Orange Balsam'), 3–6
Lime geranium (*Pelargonium nervosum*), 3–6
Lemongrass (*Cymbopogon citratus*), 1 clump
Cherry pie heliotrope (*Heliotropium arborescens*), 3–6

*The number following the botanic name indicates quantity of plants needed.

OVAL PERENNIAL GARDEN IN LILAC AND WHITE

This small (10- by 5-foot), low-maintenance garden of hardy perennial herbs provides a beautiful, summertime focal point in the middle of a lawn. It's full of deliciously scented plants with white or purple flowers. The shrub or rambling rose at the center and the edging of winter savory delineate its shape even when the rest of the plants are not at their loveliest. Best of all, there are plenty of useful plants for making potpourri and cleaning supplies. Dig the soapwort root for cleaning textiles, cut and dry the sweet woodruff for a vanilla-scented fixative, and when the Florentine iris needs to be divided, the extra rhizomes can be cleaned, sliced, dried, and cured (for two years) as a violet-scented potpourri fixative.

Maintenance. Site the garden with the lavender along the south side and the sweet woodruff on the north or northeast side, where it will be in shade. Provide a trellis or other support if you use a rambling rose rather than a shrub rose. If the area is dry, keep a soaker hose in the sweet woodruff to provide the moisture it needs, and if the soil is alkaline, acidify to pH 5.0 by adding powdered agricultural sulfur or a fertilizer containing ammonium sulfate. In the first two years after the garden is planted, it may be necessary to fill in the open spaces with pansies, violas, white marigolds, and other annuals.

Other options. If you have the space, give the bed a triple border and provide yourself with more cleaning materials by adding a band of thyme in front of the savory and one of lavender behind it. The insect-chasing lavender cotton *(Santolina chamaecyparissus)*, which looks like gray coral, makes a very interesting edging in areas where temperatures never fall below 0°F. It's prone to crown rot so be sure it has good drainage. Also, it has bright yellow, buttonlike flowers that you'll want to clip, as they don't fit the color theme. If you live in a climate with cool summers, tuck Johnny-jump-ups *(Viola tricolor)* here and there to provide more color, especially at the south-facing front of the bed, in front of the clump of lavenders, or plant an entire ribbon of it in front of the winter savory. Eat the flowers in salads or press and save them to add color to potpourri.

Oval Perennial Garden in Lilac and White

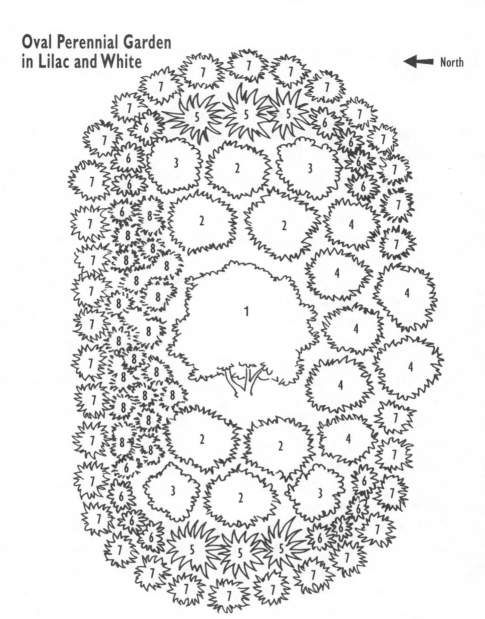

North →

1. Fragrant white shrub rose or rambling rose (Rosa spp.), 1*
2. Anise hyssop (Agastache foeniculum), 6
3. Wild bergamot (Monarda fistulosa), 4
4. Lavender (Lavandula angustifolia) or lavandin (Lavandula x intermedia), 7
5. Florentine iris (Iris germanica var. florentina), 6 clumps
6. Soapwort (Saponaria officinalis), 16
7. Winter savory (Satureja montana), 30–35
8. Sweet woodruff (Galium odoratum), 19

*The number after the botanic name indicates quantity of plants needed.

A GARDEN OF SWEET SCENTS

This curving border (10- by 5-foot) for the south wall of a house is close to my heart, being an adaptation of the garden on the protected side of my own home. It's a relatively low-maintenance garden composed primarily of hardy perennials, with a smattering of plants like anise, chamomile, and sweet Annie that can be direct-sown, and just one plant, lemon basil, that you must start indoors or keep as a potted tender perennial.

Site the garden along the south face of a structure with climbing supports for the roses, or if you have room for a wider border, purchase shrub roses and allow them to spread to their full diameter, like southern belles in hoop skirts. You can also double the length of the border by repeating the planting layout as a mirror image, starting at the costmary on the west side of the garden. For the roses, select varieties with white, yellow, or lavender flowers that bloom recurrently through the season. The Garden of Sweet Scents is at its most beautiful in summer. However, the edging of lemon thyme and the backdrop of rose canes provide some structure to the garden in other months.

Winter care. The basil is a tender perennial, which will need to be wintered indoors in cold areas. Plant it in a pot that you can sink into the soil and lift out easily at the end of the season. Scented geraniums would be a lovely addition to this garden if you have space to tuck them into, or grow them in place of anise or chamomile.

Maintenance. During the first two years after the garden is planted, it may be necessary to fill in the open spaces with pansies, violas, calendula, chervil, marjoram, borage, and other annuals. Once established, this garden requires very little aside from a bit of weeding, a heavy mulch, annual pruning of the roses after December, and a covering of straw or leaves for the roses and lavenders during the winter. Thread a soaker hose through the mints and roses to provide moisture during extended dry periods. Also, harvest the sweet Annie before it seeds if you don't want volunteers in all the wrong places. Other than that, all you need to do is harvest and inhale all the delicious scents.

A Garden of Sweet Scents

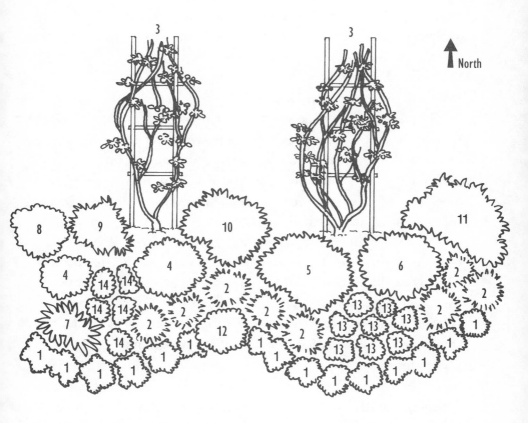

1. **Lemon thyme** *(Thymus citriodorus)*, **15***
2. **Lavender** *(Lavandula angustifolia)*, **8**
3. **Climbing, shrub, or pillar rose**
   (Rosa spp.), **2**
4. **Lemon balm** *(Melissa officinalis)*, **2**
5. **Anise hyssop** *(Agastache foeniculum)*, **1**
6. **Lemon bee balm** *(Monarda citriodora)*, **1**
7. **Florentine iris** *(Iris germanica var.*
   florentina), **1 clump**
8. **Costmary** *(Tanacetum balsamita)*, **1**

9. **Sweet Annie** *(Artemisia annua)*, **1**
10. **Spearmint** *(Mentha spicata)* **or orangemint**
    (M. x piperita 'Orange')*, **1 clump**
11. **Peppermint** *(Mentha x piperata)* **or lemon
    mint** *(Mentha x piperita var. citrata)*,
    1 clump
12. **Lemon basil** *(Ocimum basilicum var.*
    citriodorum), **1**
13. **Chamomile** *(Matricaria recutita)*, **8**
14. **Anise** *(Pimpinella anisum)*, **5**

The number after the botanic name indicates quantity of plants needed.

PEST-REPELLENT GARDEN

This corner, L-shaped shrub and perennial border will provide plenty of material for making pest-repellent sprays, cleaning supplies, sachets, and potpourri. You can site it to delineate a property boundary, to add interest to the intersection of two fences, or with one of its legs running along the south wall of a building.

The back edge of the garden is composed of a number of *Artemisia* species, so a pathway of stepping-stones and a tiny patio are used to separate these plants, with their growth-inhibiting chemical artemisin, from other plants.

Mugwort

The patio provides space for a potted bay tree, which makes a lovely focal point. Although bay trees grow 40 to 60 feet tall in their native habitats, container-grown plants seldom grow taller than 6 feet; and placed on the north or west side of the garden, the plant is unlikely to shade its neighbors. Allow the yarrow to spread between the stepping stones if it can tolerate the artemisin from the artemisias. Potted rosemary creates interest at the ends of the L. You could also include a potted patchouli, if you have room.

Other options. If you have a very wet area for them (or if you're willing to keep them watered), plant one or two large clumps of calamus. Southern gardeners can substitute various tropical salvias, such as fruit-scented and pineapple sage, for some of the plants listed here, and edge the garden with gray santolina if they prefer it to thyme, thus providing the border with gray plants at both front and rear. Northern gardeners can substitute pretty, blue-gray rue with its uniquely shaped leaves. Substitute a patchouli for the bay if you like. In cold areas, plant the tender perennials in pots and sink them into the soil. You can then easily lift them out to overwinter indoors.

Maintenance. During the first two years after the garden is planted, you may have to fill in the open spaces with marigolds, calendulas, chervil, summer savory, marjoram, borage, and other annuals. After that, you'll be so busy cutting everything back and using the trimmings that you won't have room for annuals!

Pest-Repellent Garden

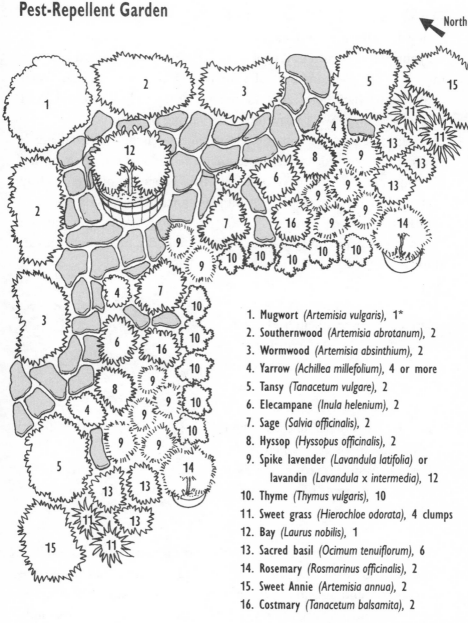

North

1. Mugwort *(Artemisia vulgaris)*, 1*
2. Southernwood *(Artemisia abrotanum)*, 2
3. Wormwood *(Artemisia absinthium)*, 2
4. Yarrow *(Achillea millefolium)*, 4 or more
5. Tansy *(Tanacetum vulgare)*, 2
6. Elecampane *(Inula helenium)*, 2
7. Sage *(Salvia officinalis)*, 2
8. Hyssop *(Hyssopus officinalis)*, 2
9. Spike lavender *(Lavandula latifolia)* or
   lavandin *(Lavandula x intermedia)*, 12
10. Thyme *(Thymus vulgaris)*, 10
11. Sweet grass *(Hierochloe odorata)*, 4 clumps
12. Bay *(Laurus nobilis)*, 1
13. Sacred basil *(Ocimum tenuiflorum)*, 6
14. Rosemary *(Rosmarinus officinalis)*, 2
15. Sweet Annie *(Artemisia annua)*, 2
16. Costmary *(Tanacetum balsamita)*, 2

*The number after the botanic name indicates quantity of plants needed.

HARVESTING THE BOUNTY

Enjoy an early-morning walk through the garden every day to check on your plants' health and condition. This is not only a real pleasure but also an important part of your herb-gardening routine. You'll soon know which herbs are budding and ready to be harvested. And frequently, such a walk turns into a harvesting session.

Cutting. A long-bladed pair of dressmaker's scissors makes it much easier, and faster, to harvest large quantities of small, multistemmed plants like thyme and lavender. Clean the scissors and oil them lightly with mineral oil after use to prevent plant juice from causing rust.

Gathering. When you cut flowers for arrangements, you put the stems into water as quickly as possible. With herbs, on the other hand, since you'll be drying the leaves, you can harvest them right into a basket. (If it has rained and the plants are dirty, I use a colander.) I carry a laundry basket when I have a lot of harvesting to do all at once, even if I'm getting different plants. I just lay the stems at right angles to each other in layers. This makes it easy to separate them when I'm ready to use them or dry them.

Use a flat basket when cutting herbs.

Digging. A spade with a narrow blade and a flat edge is handy for digging up the roots of plants without disturbing nearby plants.

PERFECT TIMING

Harvest above-ground crops in the morning, when they are full of the energy generated by their roots during the dark, and before the sun exhausts and dehydrates them. Flowers should be gathered just as they break bud. They're often perfect in the morning before marauding insects pollinate them, beginning a series of changes that destroy the flowers' form and color. On the other hand, dig root crops at twilight, when leaves have sent their energy down into the root for the night. Of course, I ignore these rules when a storm is about to break.

Rain can shred flowers, splatter gritty dirt onto plants, and dilute plant saps, so when I hear the sound of thunder I run out to the garden and start harvesting no matter what time of the day it is.

Annuals. You can harvest all annuals grown for flowers or leaves throughout the summer, as you pinch them back to shape them.

Perennials. Pinch back newly planted perennials to shape them, but don't harvest them until they've reached their full size, which may be two or three years after planting. Harvest the top half to two-thirds of the mature plant as it comes into bud. Never harvest the stem below the last set of leaves, but leave one or two sets of leaves on the lower parts of each stem so the plant will develop side shoots. Without leaves plants are extremely vulnerable to environmental stresses like heat and lack of water.

Harvest herbs above two sets of leaves.

Root crops. The usual time to harvest crops grown for their roots, like soapwort, yucca, calamus, and elecampane, is autumn, when leaves have died back. If the plants are crowded, you may want to dig them earlier, right after flowers have bloomed and withered. Dig them up, divide them, replant half, and process the rest. It's helpful to have a bucket of water in the garden to pop the roots into after shaking off the loose soil. It will soak off the worst dirt, and then the roots can be brought inside, scrubbed clean with a wire brush, peeled (if desired), and sliced or shredded for immediate use or for drying.

Seeds. Seeds like anise should be gathered when they are fully formed but still green. Cut the stems, bundle them together with a rubber band, and hang them upside down inside a paper bag, which will collect those that shatter and fall from the seed head.

Putting Down Roots

To get the strongest root production, cut off all flowering stems as soon as the plant generates them.

STORING YOUR HERBAL HARVEST

By following the suggestions in this section for preparing and storing your harvest, you can extend the shelf life of your herbs noticeably. Expect dried leaves and flowers to be good for about a year. Seeds, roots, and barks may last up to three years. Even so, I try to use most herbs within a year of harvest or purchase, in order to make room on my shelves for the new crop.

Give plants a vigorous shake outdoors as you cut them to get rid of small insects. Badly infested or dirty plants must be washed. Afterward, lay them on a cloth to dry out a bit, or spin small quantities in a salad spinner. This is the time to "garble" your harvested plants, which means to pick them over after washing and discard any inferior, damaged, or moldy parts.

HOW TO DETERMINE YOUR PROCESSING TECHNIQUE

Once the harvest is in, you must decide whether you want to use your herbs fresh or to dry and store them for the future. Ask yourself how you want to use each herb: Will you infuse it, either fresh or dried, in water? Or will you extract it in alcohol, ammonia, vinegar, glycerin, or oil? For fresh infusions, coarsely chop herbs and pour boiling water over them immediately (see pages 19–20).

Drying herb leaves and flowers for infusions and decoctions. If you plan to dry your herbs for later use in infusions or decoctions, either chop them coarsely and spread them on a drying rack or bundle them and hang them upside down for drying. The two most important criteria for successful drying are darkness and fresh air. Be sure to keep them away from direct sunlight, and choose a cool location with good air circulation; use a fan, if necessary.

Drying herb leaves and flowers for extractions. If you want to use your herbs in extractions, you can use either fresh or dried material. Each has its pros and cons: Fresh plant materials often have subtle powers lacking in dried herbs. On the other hand, the water in their tissues dilutes the liquid in which you extract them. In contrast, dried herbs are tremendously more potent, but they often lack subtlety.

You can get around this dilemma with a compromise: First, spread out the herbs on a drying rack either indoors or in the shade for about 24 hours. Some of their water will evaporate, but because they aren't completely dry, the herbs will have some beneficial qualities of both fresh and dried herbs.

Drying roots. Because of the length of time it takes for fresh roots to dry, they are more likely to become contaminated with microorganisms than are other parts of the herbs. You can use them fresh, but if you need to dry them, slice them. If high humidity is a problem in your area, grate them as fine as possible for quicker drying. Of course, grating roots exposes more surface area to contamination, so keep a fan circulating air around them as they dry. Use a fruit-and-vegetable dehydrator for drying dense roots and barks, if possible.

Not all roots need the same preparation. For instance, you must peel elecampane before drying it. On the other hand, calamus should not be peeled, because the peel contains much of the essential oil. Peeling is optional for orris, soapwort, and yucca.

Quick Drying Trick

Scatter a strand of miniature Christmas-tree lights around herbs on a drying rack. The tiny bulbs produce much less light and heat than a regular light bulb would, but provide just enough warmth to keep humidity down. Be sure to also use a fan to keep air circulating (but not directed right at the herbs) when using this method.

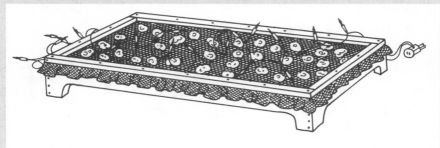

CHOOSING A PLACE TO DRY HERBS

A cool, dark, dry, paved cellar is the best place to dry herbs thoroughly and quickly. A dark, *dank* cellar is a disaster, because it allows common contaminants, including bacteria, yeasts, molds, and even *E. coli,* enterobacteria, and salmonella, to flourish.

When the harvest is rolling in and space for drying runs short, you may need to use some creativity to improvise the perfect spot to dry your herbs. Here are some suggestions to get you started:

Use a paper clip as a hook.

- Make small bunches of herbs and fasten them together with rubber bands, which contract as the herbs dry.
- Slip an S-hook or opened-out paper clip through the rubber band on the bundle, then hook the other end over the line or rack. You'll appreciate how this speeds your work.
- Attach bundled herbs to folding wooden clothes-drying racks or a clothesline strung up in your attic, if it isn't too hot.
- Hang bundles of herbs wherever you find a likely protrusion. I've used the cranks on my casement windows and even doorknobs.
- Put semidry herbs in a pillowcase and use your clothes dryer (set on "air only") to complete the process. In *Potpourri, Incense, and Other Fragrant Concoctions,* Ann Tucker Fettner confesses that she once did this during a prolonged rainy period.
- String plastic netting across a room or staple it to 1×2s (cut out at the bottom, as shown below, to increase circulation). Internet, Incorporated (see page 146) sells food-safe, FDA-approved plastic netting by the linear foot; it comes in 3-foot-wide rolls. You can use cheesecloth in the same manner, but the plastic netting is more rigid.

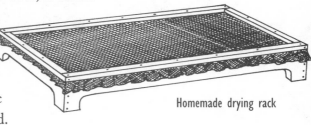

Homemade drying rack

STORING YOUR HERBS

Herbs are dry when leaves and flowers crackle to smaller pieces as you rub them between your thumb and forefinger, and stems snap easily when you break them. I usually try biting a bit of root between my front teeth to check the dryness of denser materials. For the highest-quality extractions, begin the process immediately upon drying.

It's important to store dried herbs in a cool, dry, dark place in tightly-sealed glass jars because light, heat, and humidity all affect herbs adversely. In addition, I've noticed that insect outbreaks are much more likely when jars are exposed to light and temperatures above 60°F. And the warmer it is, the more likely hatching will occur. In addition to light, temperature, and humidity, the size and quality of the herb also determine how well it will last in storage.

Warding off insects. If you think there's any possibility of insect infestation, place the bottled herbs in a freezer overnight to kill any live bugs. Or give them a 2-week stay in the freezer to render eggs harmless as well. For all herbs except fixatives (which would pick up the aromas), consider placing bay leaves and/or black peppercorns in with your herbs to deter insect pests (see pages 32–33).

Light. Light speeds up chemical processes that degrade the quality of stored herbs, which eventually makes them utterly useless for household purposes. Older herbs, especially those of flower and leaf origin, often have a faded look, a sure sign the product has lost quality.

Temperature. Max Wichtl, in *Herbal Drugs and Phytopharmaceuticals,* reports that as long ago as 1884, scientists determined that every 10-degree C (18-degree F) rise in temperature causes a doubling in the reaction rate of chemical processes, which includes the degradation of herbs. Volatile essential oils, especially, are rapidly diminished or damaged by increases in temperature. Ideally, store dried herbs at or just above freezing, and refrigerate essential oils.

Humidity. Herbs stored in the open air, in plastic containers, or in wooden drawers pick up moisture from the air. Moisture in turn activates enzymes that weaken an herb's active components. Microorganisms are also more likely to contaminate herbs when the relative humidity is higher than 60 percent.

Size of the processed herb. The smaller the pieces of herb, the more surface area is exposed to the damaging environmental effects of light, heat, moisture, as well as microorganisms, so safe storage is a must.

Quality of the herb. Much research cited in Wichtl's book has shown that aromatic herbs containing essential oils must be stored in glass, never in plastic, which not only sets up a chemical reaction with the herb, but also allows volatile oils to diffuse through it. You can also use food-safe metal tins, which exclude light. Stainless-steel or tea canisters or metal tins sold for homemade food items all are appropriate. Refrigerating or freezing herbs is an acceptable method of long-term storage, but you must protect herbs from freezer burn and moisture accumulation. Glass bottles and jars make the best storage containers for freezing.

A FINAL THOUGHT

Quality is not as crucial for herbs intended for housecleaning uses as it is for those used in medicine or cooking. When the quality of one of my aromatic herbs slips due to age or improper storage, I immediately use it to make products for household use, rather than for consumption.

CHAPTER 5

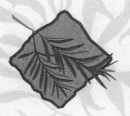

HERBAL
Housekeeping Recipes

Making your own housekeeping formulas is simple, easy, and rewarding. When you use the scents of your favorite herbs and essential oils, you'll find that your most tedious chores are almost sublime — or at least, they're more enjoyable than working with chemically scented products. The herbs and essential oils add much more than fragrance, too. They actually cut greases, attract dust, fight bacteria, and stimulate the immune system, naturally, while lifting your spirits as you work. I recommend my favorite herbs and essential oils for making these products, but you may find others that work equally well. As you become more experienced, you'll find it's easy to substitute your own favorites for those used here.

In this chapter you'll find recipes for all of your household cleaning needs, from laundry soaps to kitchen and bathroom cleaners to safe and gentle products for the nursery. There are heavy-duty scouring powders to get the soap scum and mineral stains out of porcelain fixtures; sweet-smelling, nontoxic cleaners to wash kitchen counters and children's rooms; metal polishes and leather cleaners and restorers; carpet cleaners and wood furniture creams; spot removers, laundry detergents, and insect pest deterrents; and, finally, an assortment of herb crafts to scent your linens, chase away fabric-damaging moths, sweeten up your shoes, and refresh and cleanse the air in the whole house.

You'll want to refer to Chapter 2, Supplies and Methods, for complete directions on how to prepare infusions, extractions, and other basic techniques that are part of these recipes. And examine the charts on herbal housekeeping ingredients, essential oils, and fixatives, beginning on page 136, for information about any unfamiliar ingredients in these recipes. The charts describe these ingredients and tell you where you can purchase them. I hope you will enjoy using these formulas and perhaps experiment with your own adaptations to make all of your housekeeping jobs more enjoyable and your whole home looking — and smelling — its very best.

SCOURING POWDERS

Use scouring powders, along with a helping of elbow grease, to remove tough grime on hard surfaces like counter tops, porcelain fixtures, and wall tile. The essential oils speed things up by dissolving greasy dirt and disinfecting surfaces. Scouring powders vary in abrasiveness depending on which minerals (such as chalk, baking soda, borax, salt, or washing soda) you use. If you prefer soft scrubbers, each recipe explains how to make a paste variation.

Storage. Store the powders in a metal or glass shaker, sealing holes with aluminum foil to prevent the oils from evaporating between uses. (See Super Shakers on page 91 for storage ideas.)

Low-Abrasion Scouring Powder

Low-abrasion formulas are safe for fiberglass and the plastics used in appliances. This recipe and those that follow can be modified to make an easy-to-use paste by adding liquid soap to the powder.

1 ½ cups chalk
4–4½ teaspoons essential oils (see below for suggestions)

1. Wearing a dust mask, place the chalk in a bowl. Add the essential oils. Using a wire whisk, thoroughly blend the oils into the powder.
2. Apply with a dampened sponge, or for more abrasive power, use a loofah, ayate cloth (a coarse natural-fiber scrubber), or Teflon scrubber pad.

PERSONAL FAVORITES

Bracing Fresh Air: 2 teaspoons lavender oil, 1½ teaspoons spruce or fir oil, and ½ teaspoon eucalyptus oil

Citrus Scrubber: 1½ teaspoons each grapefruit, lemon, and orange oils. If you prefer, use tangerine oil in place of any or all of these citrus oils.

Low-Abrasion Soft Scrubber Paste

To make a soft scrubber paste, add ¾ cup liquid soap (such as Dr. Bronner's Liquid Lavender Castile Soap) to the Low-Abrasion Scouring Powder.

Gentle Scouring Powder

Use this scouring powder to remove greasy dirt from appliances, porcelain fixtures, tile floors, and stainless-steel sinks. The baking soda, while gentle, is a bit more abrasive than the low-abrasion chalk formula on page 91.

> 1½ cups baking soda
> 4½ teaspoons essential oils (see below for suggestions)

1. Wearing a dust mask, place the baking soda in a bowl. Add the essential oils, and use a wire whisk to blend them thoroughly into the powder.
2. Apply with a dampened sponge, or for more abrasive power, use a loofah, ayate cloth, or Teflon scrubber pad.

PERSONAL FAVORITES

Citrus and Mint: 1 tablespoon tangerine essential oil and 1 teaspoon spearmint essential oil

Lavender and Rosemary: 1 tablespoon lavender essential oil and 1 teaspoon rosemary essential oil

Gentle Soft Scrubber

For a light- to medium-duty soft scrubber, add ¾ cup liquid soap (such as Dr. Bronner's Liquid Lavender Castile Soap) to the basic powder. Use a funnel to get the mixture into a plastic squeeze bottle. Be sure to label clearly, as it looks a bit like cake frosting.

Heavy-Duty Scouring Powder

Use this heavy-duty scouring powder on dirty or stained toilets, tubs, ovens, and nonaluminum pots and pans. Avoid getting this powder on grout, however, as the washing soda may react with the grout and weaken it.

> ½ cup baking soda
> ½ cup borax
> ½ cup washing soda
> 4½ teaspoons essential oils (see page 93 for suggestions)

1. Wearing a dust mask, combine baking soda, borax, and washing soda in bowl. Add the essential oils, and using a whisk, blend the oils thoroughly into the powder.
2. Apply with a sponge; for more abrasive power, use a loofah, ayate cloth, or Teflon scrubber pad.

PERSONAL FAVORITE
Minty-Fresh Blend: 1 tablespoon peppermint oil, 1 teaspoon anise oil, and ½ teaspoon clove oil

Heavy-Duty Scrubber Paste

For a heavy-duty scrubber paste, add ¾ to 1 cup liquid soap (such as Dr. Bronner's Liquid Peppermint Castile Soap). Be sure to label the container; this mixture looks just like grated Parmesan cheese!

Toilet Bowl Cleaner

To make a toilet bowl cleaner out of the Gentle Scouring Powder (page 92), sprinkle about ½ cup of the scouring powder into the toilet, spray with any herbal vinegar to create a bubbling paste, and use a brush to scour. Or, sprinkle Heavy-Duty Scouring Powder (page 92) in the toilet and leave overnight. In the morning, spray with an herbal vinegar and scrub.

Get Rid of Hard-Water Deposits

Citric acid (see page 136) will dissolve hard-water lime deposits in toilets. Sprinkle the surface generously with enough powdered citric acid to cover the surface, and scour with a brush. Spray with herbal vinegar if more moisture is needed. If this isn't strong enough to do the job, purchase powdered oxalic acid and follow the directions on the package label. You'll find oxalic acid in the grocery store cleaning aisle with the other powdered cleaners under the trade name Zud.

Heavy-Duty Spray-and-Brush Toilet Cleaner

Shake this cleaner well before each use, since the lemon essential oil tends to rise to the top. It dissolves rings and cleans up overflow messes with ease. Herbal ammonia is brown, so rinse carefully.

> 1 tablespoon lemon essential oil
> 1 teaspoon lime essential oil
> 4 tablespoons alcohol (ethyl or isopropyl)
> 1½ cups eucalyptus vinegar extraction
> 2 tablespoons liquid soap (such as Lifetree's All-Purpose Spray Cleaner)
> Up to 2 tablespoons plain or herbal ammonia

1. In a glass measuring cup, dissolve the essential oils in the alcohol.
2. Pour the mixture into a spray bottle.
3. Add the herbal vinegar, liquid soap, and herbal ammonia.
4. Shake well, then spray all surfaces of the toilet bowl, and brush to clean.

Storage. Store in a glass or plastic spray bottle, and use within 6 months. Keep away from small children.

SURFACE CLEANERS

Use the scouring powders and soft scrubbers on pages 91–93 for kitchen counter tops, appliances, painted walls, vinyl or ceramic tile, and other hard, impermeable surfaces. To clean light soil on walls, cabinets, counter tops, and floors, add 2 tablespoons of borax or 1 to 2 tablespoons of castile soap to 1 gallon of hot water or hot herb infusion.

Cleaning Marble

Use mildly alkaline soaps to wash marble, such as Essential Oil–Enhanced Liquid Castile Soap (page 95) and Essential Oil–Enhanced Murphy's Soap (page 96). Avoid vinegar solutions, because the acid can damage the surface.

Heavy-Duty Cleaner

When your cleaning tasks need a bit more power, mix up this formula. You can also use a combination of washing soda and borax, in equal amounts.

> 1–2 tablespoons essential oil (see below for suggestions)
> ½–1 cup herb-infused ammonia or ¼–½ washing soda or borax
> 1 gallon (or more) herb-infused or plain hot water

Combine essential oil with ammonia, washing soda, or borax in a bucket. Add hot water.

Storage. Use mixture immediately.

PERSONAL FAVORITES
General: Lavender essential oil
Flea control: Orange essential oil
Disinfecting and energizing: Peppermint essential oil

Herbal Vinegar to the Rescue

To disinfect, spray herbal vinegar or alcohol extractions directly on surfaces, leave on for at least 10 minutes, then wipe off. Or, use ¼ cup vinegar or alcohol in 1 gallon of rinse water.

Essential Oil–Enhanced Liquid Castile Soap

The glycerin in this formula acts as a solvent for the essential oil; it is also an emulsifier, blending the essential oil and the soap. Dilute this product to clean fine hand-washables, counter tops, lightly soiled walls, floors, and fixtures. It's very safe and nontoxic.

> 1 tablespoon essential oil (see page 96 for suggestions)
> 1 tablespoon glycerin
> 1 cup scented or unscented Dr. Bronner's Liquid Castile Soap

1. Combine the essential oil with the glycerin in a small bowl. Blend them thoroughly before adding the mixture to the soap. Adding essential oil to liquid soap without glycerin causes curdling.
2. Add the essential oil and glycerin mixture to the soap. Stir well to blend. Pour into a labeled glass or plastic bottle.

Use. Add 1 tablespoon to a basin of warm water for fine hand-washables, or ¼ cup or more to machine wash. Use ¼ to 1 cup of herbal vinegar in the rinse water to remove soap residue.

Storage. Store in a glass jar for a year or more, or in plastic for 6 months to 1 year.

PERSONAL FAVORITES

Orange, tangerine, lemon, grapefruit, fir, spruce, and lavender are all good choices and relatively inexpensive essential oils, although you can try more expensive ones, as well.

Essential Oil-Enhanced Murphy's Soap

This is my favorite soap for cleaning semipermeable surfaces like wood floors, painted walls, shellacked woodwork, and varnished furniture. Its ability to clean and disinfect is enhanced when essential oils are added. For woodwork and furniture, I like to complete the job with Duster's Delight (page 104).

> 4 cups Murphy's Oil Soap Concentrate
> (available at paint stores)
> 8 tablespoons essential oil (see below for suggestions)

1. Measure the soap concentrate into a glass jar.

2. Add essential oils and beat thoroughly with a paddle or flat spoon to disperse them completely.

Use. Add about 1 tablespoon of the mixture to a quart of hot, strained herb infusion. Whisk to a froth. Apply with a sponge or soft cloth. Rinse with ½ cup herbal vinegar in 1 gallon water (for woodwork, I like citrus peel vinegar). Wipe dry if you follow this treatment with Duster's Delight.

Storage. Store concentrate in a glass jar for a year or more.

PERSONAL FAVORITE

5 tablespoons lavender essential oil, 2 tablespoons orange essential oil, and 1 tablespoon rosemary essential oil

GLASS CLEANERS

Window-washing equipment is standard fare: a spray bottle for the solution, lots of huck toweling or other lint-free cotton or linen rags (like old dish towels or cotton-knit T-shirts) to clean with, and a chamois or clean, dry cloths for the final polish. Here are some tips to make your work go more efficiently:

- To avoid the streaks caused when the sun dries the solution before you have a chance to rub it off, wash windows on overcast days (or, on sunny days, work on the shady side of the house).
- It's best to work with a partner, so one of you can work inside and one outside. If the outside partner uses only vertical strokes and the inside partner uses only horizontal strokes, it will be easy to figure out which side is streaked and needs more polishing.
- Keep a sharp scraper handy to deal with dried paint, tape residue, insect spots, and other tough grime.

Herbal Vinegar Window and Mirror Wash

For sparkling clean windows, vinegar solutions have no equal. If you use herb infusions with insect-repellent qualities, you'll discourage flies and mosquitoes from clustering at your windows.

> 3 cups water
> ¼ cup, plus 2 tablespoons herbal vinegar, strained
> (see below for suggestions)

Pour the water into a spray bottle. Add herbal vinegar. Shake well. Label.
Use. Spray on windows, then polish with a clean, dry cloth.
Storage. Store in a spray bottle. Keeps for about 6 months.

PERSONAL FAVORITES

Fragrant herbs: Anise hyssop, basil, bay, eucalyptus, hyssop, lavender, marjoram, oregano, rosemary, roses, sage, sweet Annie, sweet grass, winter savory

Bug-repellent herbs: Epazoté, southernwood, sweet Annie, tansy, wormwood, yarrow

Window Screens

Wash screens with an herbal castile soap or Essential Oil–Enhanced Murphy's Soap (see page 96), and allow to dry. Spray with a bug-repellent herb infusion made with any of the following herbs: bay, bee balm, calamus, epazoté, ginkgo, hyssop, mugwort, sage, southernwood, sweet Annie, sweet grass, tansy, wormwood, or yarrow.

You can also use a diluted herbal isopropyl alcohol for this, but try a test area before spraying the entire screen, to make sure it doesn't damage the screening material.

Glass Scratch Remover

Sometimes fine scratches mar your windows and mirrors, even when they're sparkling clean. Try this scratch remover for fine scratches. If you have a deep scratch, try Cerium Oxide Polishing Powder (for suppliers, see "Glaziers," in your Yellow Pages).

> 1 tablespoon herb infusion
> 1 tablespoon plain glycerin or herbal glycerate
> 1–2 tablespoons powdered chalk

1. Combine the herb infusion with the glycerin in a small bowl.
2. Add drops of the liquid to the powdered chalk, stirring until a thick paste forms. (You may not need all the liquid.)

Use. Apply with a soft cloth, burnishing at right angles to scratch. Rinse. Repeat if needed. This formula is intended for immediate use.

METAL POLISHES

Lustrous, glowing metals are attractive, welcoming elements of every gracious home. The nontoxic polishes in this section will have you smiling happily while you bring a bright glowing sheen to brass, silver, and other household metals.

Aluminum Polish

To clean the inside of an aluminum pan, pour any undiluted herb vinegar into it, and simmer over low heat for 10–60 minutes, until all discoloration disappears. Discard the vinegar afterward. To clean small aluminum items, put them in a saucepan, cover them with herb vinegar, and simmer over low heat until they are clean. (Use aluminum, enameled steel, enameled cast-iron, or stainless-steel pans for this purpose. Do not use cast iron, which reacts with the vinegar, not only interfering with the cleaning process, but affecting the seasoning of the pan, as well.)

Paste-style aluminum polish. For non-submersible items or for extra power, mix about ¼ cup citric acid with enough herbal vinegar to create a sticky paste, and rub on. (Don't use baking soda or washing soda solutions to clean aluminum as they will dull it.)

Brass Polish

Clean lacquered brass with mild soap and water. For unlacquered brass, dampen the object with vinegar (or equal parts of vinegar and isopropyl alcohol), sprinkle with salt, and scour with a Teflon-safe abrasive pad moistened with vinegar. Add more salt, if needed.

Paste-style brass polish. Combine ¼ cup chalk with enough herbal vinegar to make a paste. For more acidity, blend 1–2 tablespoons citric acid with the chalk, or combine Gentle Soft Scrubber (page 92) with herb-infused isopropyl alcohol.

Chrome and Stainless-Steel Polish

Use herb vinegar or herb-infused isopropyl alcohol to clean all chrome and stainless steel. This is especially good for cleaning car chrome in the winter, as it doesn't freeze.

Paste-style chrome and stainless-steel polish. For mild abrasion, mix ¼ cup chalk with enough alcohol to create a sticky paste. (As alcohol prevents water spotting, it's better than vinegar for use on chrome. To get rid of soap scum, however, combine chalk with vinegar, or use vinegar alone.) Or, use Low-Abrasion Soft Scrubber Paste (page 91).

Copper Polish

Dampen the copper item, sprinkle it with salt, and then spray with any herbal vinegar, especially citrus peel vinegar. Rub with an abrasive pad or the cut surface of half a lemon or lime. (Lime is more acidic than lemon, so it works faster). Rinse well and dry.

Silver Polish

Low-Abrasion Soft Scrubber Paste (page 91) made with Bracing Fresh Air essential oils makes a wonderful silver polish. Apply with a soft cloth or chamois. Rinse well and dry immediately. Gentle Soft Scrubber (page 92) works almost as well.

CARPET AND RUG CLEANERS

Carpets and rugs are soft underfoot and muffle sounds, making our homes quiet refuges from the outer world. Unfortunately, they also attract and hold dust, dirt, odors, and microorganisms, all of which exacerbate allergies. The recipes in this section are designed to deodorize carpeting, remove stains, and discourage fleas and other insects.

Herb-and-Baking Soda Refresher

This herbal powder whisks away odors from carpets. Purchase powdered herbs, or pulverize herbs in a coffee grinder or spice mill. (Clean the coffee mill first by whirling dry bread crumbs in it, and discard the first batch of herbs if they smell of coffee.) For light-colored carpets, use ½ tablespoon of essential oil per 1 cup of baking soda instead of herbs, or use crumbled rather than powdered herbs. If the carpeting smells very bad, pretreat before using this refresher. First, remove any stains (see Essential-Oil Ammonia Treatment for Carpets on page 101, and Rosemary and Fuller's Earth Grease Remover on page 116), then use powdered zeolite according to the package directions.

2½ cups each powdered roses, powdered lavender, powdered rosemary, and powdered sandalwood

10 cups baking soda

1. Blend all the ingredients together thoroughly.
2. Vacuum the rug, then sprinkle refresher onto the carpet and spread it with a natural bristle brush. Leave it overnight or for several days, then vacuum. Avoid walking on the carpet during treatment.

Essential Oil-Ammonia Treatment for Carpets

Full-strength orange or rosemary essential oils remove grease from wool carpeting. For other stains, make this ammonia-essential oil formula. Although the solution, as well as undiluted essential oils, is safe for wool carpets, it may damage the carpet padding, so place an absorbent pad between the carpet and foam pad before treating, if possible. If the carpet is made from synthetic fibers, check with the manufacturer or test an unobtrusive area before treating. For stain removal, use regular ammonia rather than herb-infused ammonia, which may discolor the carpet.

Safety first. Open a window for ventilation during this treatment.

> ½–4 tablespoons orange or rosemary essential oil
> 1 cup ammonia
> 1 cup cool water

1. Combine the essential oil, ammonia, and water in a glass spray bottle. Shake well.
2. Place an absorbent cloth between the carpet and carpet pad, directly under the stain.
3. Spray the stain heavily, then dab with another absorbent cloth to pick up the stain residue. Continue spraying and dabbing until the stain is gone. (Shake the solution vigorously before each application.)
4. Remove the absorbent cloth from between the carpet and carpet pad, and replace it with a clean dry cloth.
5. Sprinkle bentonite (see page 136), borax, or baking soda on the spot to absorb any remaining liquid. Allow the powder to sit on the carpet until it is completely dry, then vacuum the residue. Avoid walking on the treated area until it has been vacuumed. Remove the cloth from under the treated area.

Orange Peel and Borax Solution

If you have animals, you may have fleas lurking about on floors, car-peting, and upholstery. For effective flea removal, you must concur-rently treat as many surfaces as possible, including bare floors and carpeting, as well as the upholstered surfaces in the area. Vacuum or sweep all floors, then mop non-carpeted floors with this Orange Peel and Borax Solution. Next, treat all carpeted and upholstered surfaces with Orange Peel and Boric Acid Treatment for Fleas (below).

Safety first. If you are pregnant, do not use essential oil of pennyroyal.

> 1–4 tablespoons orange essential oil
> 1 cup borax
> 2 gallons hot pennyroyal infusion or hot water

Combine all ingredients in a 3-gallon bucket.

Use. Mop all bare floors. Instead of rinsing, make a second batch of the solution and go over the floors once again. The residue of invisi-bly fine borax crystals will further deter the insects.

Orange Peel and Boric Acid Treatment for Fleas

To make this flea treatment even more effective, add ¼–1 pound of diatomaceous earth to the powder. This powder is intended to be left in place, except on carpets (both boric acid and diatomaceous earth can damage fibers) and in high traffic areas.

> 1 pound granulated orange peel
> 1 pound boric acid
> ¼ pound powdered calamus root
> ¼ pound powdered painted daisy (pyrethrum daisy) flower buds
> 1 ounce orange essential oil (optional)

1. Vacuum the area to be treated.
2. Combine the orange peel, boric acid, calamus root, and flower buds. Stir in the orange essential oil, if desired.
3. *For flea control,* sprinkle under couch cushions, on carpeting under furniture, along baseboards, under beds, between mattresses and

box springs, and anywhere fleas may be hiding. *For roach control,* put some under the kitchen sink, inside cabinets, and on pantry shelves. Leave overnight, then vacuum traffic areas.

Storage. Store in a carefully labelled glass jar or metal container for up to 6 months.

Safety first. Wear a dust mask while blending and applying powders containing boric acid or diatomaceous earth. Pregnant women should not use essential oil of pennyroyal. Some people develop a rash from pyrethrum flowers, so wear gloves when you work with this powder. Keep this powder away from small children.

Herbal Variation

For a strictly herbal solution, leave out the boric acid from the Orange Peel and Boric Acid recipe on page 102, and simply blend the herbs together. Use as described at the left, and also treat the area between the rug and its padding, if possible; leave the powder in place for up to 6 months.

FURNITURE AND WOODWORK CLEANERS AND POLISHES

I love the warmth and beauty of wood cabinets, moldings, and furniture, which add so much to the ambiance of a gracious, welcoming home. These cleaning formulas enhance wood's natural beauty.

Wood-Washing Formula

Use this formula to wash wood surfaces, including floors, cabinets, and woodwork, whenever they need it. The ingredients are safe enough to use weekly.

> ½ cup dried herbs, such as lemon balm, lemon thyme, sweet cicely, costmary, and/or lavender
> 1 cup water
> ½ cup Essential Oil–Enhanced Murphy's Soap (page 96)
> 1 gallon water
> ½ cup citrus peel vinegar

1. Make an infusion with the herbs, and steep for 15 minutes. Strain.
2. Add Essential Oil–Enhanced Murphy's Soap to the hot infusion, and whisk to dissolve. If the solution has cooled too much to dissolve the soap, heat the mixture in a microwave oven or double boiler. Apply the soap solution with a sponge or soft cloth.
3. In a bucket, combine 1 gallon of water with the citrus peel vinegar. Use the solution as a rinse, then wipe dry.

Using Essential Oils on Wood

Essential oils add fragrance, luster, and bacteria-bashing qualities to each of the following formulas.

Dusting Polish. Open windows wide. With a spray bottle, apply lemon, rosemary, lavender, or other essential oil to a lamb's-wool duster, and use on shellacked or varnished woodwork and furniture. Do only one room or object per day, as the fragrance is quite intense. Test before using any undiluted essential oil on painted woodwork. You can dilute by using 1¼ cups of mineral or jojoba oil to 1 tablespoon of essential oil.

Duster's Delight. Mix up to 1 tablespoon of lemon or other essential oil into ¼ cup of mineral oil, then combine with 1 cup Citra-Solv in a spray bottle. Before applying, damp-mop the surface with water and a splash of herbal vinegar. Spray a clean dust mop with Duster's Delight, and dust the surface. Lamb's-wool dusters or light-colored, recycled wool sweaters make the best mops, as they attract dust effectively.

Fragrant Oil Finish. Mix together 1½ teaspoons of balsam of Peru essential oil and 1½ teaspoons of other essential oils (such as citrus, evergreen, and lavender), then combine with 1 cup of mineral or jojoba oil. Apply to unfinished (or unvarnished, but oiled) wood furniture with soft, lint-free rags. Allow to soak in. Wipe off excess, if required. Reapply if necessary, especially to the end grain of the wood. For a more resistant finish, follow with Fragrant Wood Furniture Polish (page 105) or Fragrant Furniture and Floor Wax (page 107).

Fragrant Wood Furniture Polish

This wax with the pleasant vanilla fragrance of balsam of Peru not only protects wood surfaces, especially unfinished wood, but it's also a pleasure to use. For a stiffer wax, increase the amount of beeswax to 2 ounces. For a harder wax that can be buffed, use 1–1½ ounces paraffin or carnauba wax (see page 136) instead of the beeswax.

> 1 ounce beeswax
> 1 cup mineral or jojoba oil
> 1½ teaspoons balsam of Peru essential oil
> 1½ teaspoons other essential oils (see below for suggestions)

1. Melt the beeswax in the oil in the top of a double boiler. Remove from heat and allow to cool just until a crescent of wax forms at the edge of the pan.
2. Add balsam of Peru and other essential oils. Stir well.

Use. *For unfinished or oil-finished wood,* use this solution while it is still liquid, as this gives the best penetration. Use a paintbrush or lamb's-wool pad to apply. Rub in well and allow to cool.

For varnished or shellacked wood, apply the cooled solution with a soft, lint-free rag, then buff well.

Storage. Store excess furniture polish in a labelled glass jar indefinitely.

PERSONAL FAVORITES

Sandalwood, rosewood, balsam of tolu, tangerine, grapefruit, and lemon

Finished with Fingerprints

To eradicate fingerprints from your wood furniture, apply undiluted Essential Oil—Enhanced Murphy's Soap (page 96) directly on the area to be cleaned. Rub with a damp sponge, then rinse well. Add a splash of herbal vinegar to the rinse water for even better results.

Furniture Cream

This rich emulsion is like hand lotion for your furniture. It's a bit complicated to make, but worth the effort. The trickiest part of this process is to get the infusion and the oil/wax solution to the right temperature at the same time. If the infusion is too cold, some of the wax will precipitate out, forming gritty bits, and the emulsion won't whip up properly.

Traditionally, this furniture cream is made with a lemon balm infusion, but you can use any herb you like. If you use herb-infused oil, calendula and/or chamomile flowers are a good choice. Mineral or jojoba oils are the preferred oils, as they don't go rancid. Combine this with lemon essential oil, as it, too, prevents rancidity. This recipe makes just enough to fit in a wide-mouthed 16-ounce jar.

½ cup dried herbs (or 1 cup fresh) (see page 107 for suggestions)
1½ cups water
1 ounce cocoa butter
¾ ounce beeswax
1 cup plain or herb-infused oil (mineral, jojoba, walnut, or olive oil)
1 tablespoon essential oils (see page 107 for suggestions)

1. Make an infusion with the herbs, cover, and allow to steep while you proceed to the next step.
2. Combine the cocoa butter and beeswax with the oil in a double boiler. When the cocoa butter and beeswax have melted, remove pan from heat. Allow to cool just until a crescent of wax forms at the edge of the pan.
3. Strain 1 cup plus 1 tablespoon of the infusion into a measuring cup. Test the temperature: it should be between 95° and 105°F. If it's too cool, warm the infusion in a microwave oven. If it's too hot, allow it to cool, but set the oil solution over low heat so it doesn't skim over completely while you're waiting.
4. Pour the warm infusion into a blender. Put the lid on and turn the blender on high. With the blender on, quickly pour in the oil solution, using a funnel if necessary to direct the solution in through

the access opening in the lid. Allow the blender to run continuously while the emulsion forms. If the solution is a little too hot, it may take a bit longer.

5. Once the mixture has thickened, turn off the blender and scrape down the sides with a spatula. Allow it to cool for 15 or 20 minutes.

6. Add up to 1 tablespoon essential oils and blend again.

Use. Apply with a soft cloth, and rub to a lustrous finish.

Storage. Place in a glass jar with a lid, and label carefully. Store unused furniture cream in the refrigerator or freezer to prevent mold and rancidity. Mineral and jojoba oils keep indefinitely.

Some Like It Hot

It's better to err on the side of combining solutions that are a bit too hot, since they will emulsify as they cool, as long as you keep the blender running. This means that you may have to wait a bit longer until they get to the temperature at which the emulsion forms, but that's much better than getting a gritty or incomplete emulsion that you can't possibly salvage.

PERSONAL FAVORITES
For the infusion: Comfrey, lemon balm, sweet Cicely, lemon thyme, and/or roses
For the essential oils: Lemon essential oil with balsam of Peru or lavender and rosemary essential oils with sandalwood and/or frankincense

Fragrant Furniture and Floor Wax

Floor wax is usually made with a solvent like mineral spirits. Once applied to the wood, the solvent evaporates, leaving behind the hard wax to protect the floor or furniture. Because mineral spirits, a petroleum derivative, may cause health problems, the following recipes substitute an ingredient for the mineral spirits: Citra-Solv (a commercial product made from essential oil components) and turpentine (a volatile essential oil distilled from resin taken from coniferous trees, especially longleaf pines). If you'd like to make a harder mixture that you can buff, substitute paraffin or carnauba for the beeswax, and use 4 ounces of beeswax to 1 cup of Citra-Solv.

> 5 ounces beeswax
>
> 1 cup Citra-Solv
>
> 1 tablespoon lemon or tangerine essential oil

1. Melt the wax in a double boiler on low heat. When it has completely melted, remove from heat.
2. Add the Citra-Solv. Stir well. Allow to cool slightly.
3. Add the essential oil.
4. Carefully pour the wax into a jar. Label and allow it to cool before using. It will set up to a very soft paste.

Use. Apply with a soft cloth or lamb's-wool pad; buff. Waxing should be done only once a year. In between waxings, wash and dry-mop wood floors with Duster's Delight (page 104).

Storage. Store in a glass jar in a cool, dark place; it keeps for years.

Safe Use of Solvents

Solvents are combustible, so take these precautions with them:
- Most important, melt the wax first, remove it from the heat, and then pour in the solvent. *Never* heat the solvent. The fumes are very strong and the potential for a fire is great.
- When heating the wax, use a double boiler over a low flame.
- Keep the vent hood of your stove top running.
- Have a fire extinguisher nearby.
- Don't leave the room during the process.
- Waxy rags can spontaneously combust, so dispose of them properly. If in doubt, check with your local fire department.
- Don't machine-wash rags coated with waxes or solvents, as there's a chance that a spark from the electrical system could ignite the fumes from the solvents.

Evergreen-Scented Floor Wax

The spruce or fir essential oil in this floor wax makes your home smell like the north woods. The wax makes a firm, protective coating for your wood floors that will last for at least a year.

> 4 ounces beeswax
>
> 1 cup turpentine
>
> 1 tablespoon spruce or fir essential oil

1. Melt the wax in a double boiler on low heat. When it has completely melted, remove from heat.
2. Add the turpentine. Stir well. Allow to cool slightly.
3. Add the essential oil. Carefully pour the floor wax into a glass jar. Label and allow it to cool. It will set up to a very soft paste.

Use. Apply with a soft cloth or lamb's-wool pad; buff. Wax once a year; wash and dry-mop with Duster's Delight (page 104) weekly.

Storage. Store in a glass jar in a cool, dark place; it keeps for years.

LAUNDRY AIDS

Laundry has a lot in common with death and taxes. They all seem to be inevitable. Here are my solutions for the ever-present laundry pile. I'm sorry I can't do anything about the other two.

Delicate Fabric Froth

Yucca or soapwort roots clean fine fabrics, antique baskets, tapestries, hats, and other textiles that should not be immersed in water, as well as lightly soiled natural-fiber upholstery fabrics and Oriental rugs.

> ¼ cup powdered dry yucca root or soapwort root
>
> 3 cups water

1. Put yucca or soapwort roots in the bottom of a blender. Boil water, then pour it over the powdered roots. With the lid on the blender, run on high for 2 or 3 minutes, or until froth no longer increases. Allow mixture to settle before removing the lid. To avoid gritty roots permeating the suds, don't pour the liquid out of the blender.

2. Scoop out the froth with your hand or a soft brush, and gently rub it into textile. Allow suds to dry on the object, then brush or rinse off. If more froth is needed, blitz the liquid in blender again. When froth is gone, strain the liquid remaining in the blender, and use it to hand-wash silk and wool items, or even your hair.

Storage. Use immediately.

Dryer Scents

To scent clothes naturally, put a drop of lavender, rosemary, or any citrus essential oil on a cotton handkerchief, and toss it in the dryer near the end of the cycle.

Essential Oil–Powdered Detergent Booster

This naturally scented detergent not only smells wonderful, but the essential oil boosts your immune system as well. One detergent that works well is Arm and Hammer Perfume and Dye Free detergent.

> 2 tablespoons orange, lavender, or rosemary essential oil
> 5 pounds unscented powdered laundry detergent

Combine the essential oil with the laundry detergent in a large kettle, and mix well with a heavy-duty whisk.

Use. Use the amount (or a bit less) called for on the detergent label.

Storage. Mix and store in a large kettle with a tight-fitting lid to prevent the oils from evaporating. (Although plastic containers are convenient for storage, essential oils tend to dissipate through plastic, so glass or metal is preferred.)

Soap Residues

An herb-vinegar rinse removes residues of castile soaps, old-fashioned laundry soaps, or washing soda. Add ½–1 cup of herbal vinegar, preferably made with lavender or rosemary, to the rinse cycle.

Special Handling

Silks. Because silk is a protein fiber, it responds better to shampoo (such as Nature's Gate Original) than to detergent.
* Use warm water and the delicate cycle.
* Machine wash only a few items at a time in a full load of water.
* Rinse twice in cool water to ensure that you're rid of all the suds.
* Dry in the dryer, delicate cycle or hang-dry. Touch up lightly with a cool iron, if needed.

Wools and cashmeres. Treat these fabrics much as you would silk, except rinse them in warm water. Before storing woolens, wash, then rinse them in a moth-repellent herbal vinegar solution, like spike lavender *(Lavendula latifolia)* or southernwood.
* Separate colors scrupulously, to avoid getting light fibers on a dark sweater.
* Use warm water and the delicate cycle.
* Wash only a few items at a time in a full load of water. Woolens tend to felt if crowding forces them to rub against one another.
* Rinse in warm water. Do not "shock" wool items with temperature changes, as this, too, tends to felt wool.

Down and feathers. Wash pillows and comforters frequently to prevent allergic reactions to dust mites.
* Machine-wash using warm water and a gentle cycle.
* Use herbal shampoo or Murphy's Oil Soap (not detergent, which is too harsh).
* After the washer has filled for the final rinse, add either ½ cup plain glycerin or an extract made with glycerin and marsh mallow root *(Althaea officinalis)* or comfrey root to restore "life" to the damp feathers.
* Dry thoroughly in the dryer, not on a line. Because the dryer is quicker, mildew won't develop and the feathers get a good fluffing.

STAIN REMOVERS AND PRETREATMENTS

Essential oil of rosemary is my favorite stain remover, especially for grease spots. The rosemary-based formulas on the following pages are similar, but they use different liquids, depending on the stain. If it's more convenient to make a paste, combine the essential oil with the mineral first, then add enough liquid to make a paste.

Safety first. If you're pregnant, substitute lavender essential oil for rosemary. Rosemary contains some camphor, which is toxic, and therefore should be avoided during pregnancy.

Stain Removal Tips

- Always test formula on an inconspicuous area such as a seam or hem, especially with nonwashable fabrics.
- Blot fresh stains immediately with a clean cloth to absorb as much liquid as possible. Neutralize acid stains by sprinkling them with baking soda. Allow the baking soda to set while preparing a stain-removing solution. Vacuum or shake off baking soda before continuing the treatment.
- Start with a 3-percent solution of whatever formula you're using. If it doesn't completely remove the stain, repeat the treatment.
- If greasy dirt or stains are barely affected by the treatment, increase the amount of essential oil and/or change the carrier.
- Always use cold water when pretreating stains on fabrics. Hot water sets most stains, making them harder to remove.
- Treat acid stains, such as tomato sauce, with cold water, neutralize them with baking soda, then flush them with ammonia.
- Treat alkaline stains, such as perspiration stains, with vinegar.
- Treat greasy stains with a solvent like alcohol, glycerin, or Murphy's Oil Soap, depending on the fabric. Many stains respond to liquid detergent.
- Treat combination stains, like coffee with cream, that contain an acid, a protein, and a grease either in two steps or with a combination of two solvents.

Rosemary-Ammonia Stain Remover

Keep this simple solution handy for stains on any washable fabric that are caused by perspiration, urine, or vomit. Dilute the solution with an equal amount of water for silk or wool. Neutralize any acidity in fresh stains by blotting them first with baking soda.

½–4 tablespoons rosemary essential oil
1 cup ammonia

1. Combine the essential oil and ammonia in a glass spray bottle.
2. Shake well to combine. Because the oil and ammonia don't mix well, you'll need to continue shaking before and during use.
Storage. Store for a year or more in a labelled glass spray bottle.

Rosemary-Vinegar Stain Remover

This stain remover is useful for getting out many different kinds of spills, spots, and stains, including alcohol, beer, coffee, cola, fruit juice, tea, tomato juice/sauce, washable ink, and wine. Before treating any wet stains, sprinkle a heavy coating of baking soda over the spill, allow it to soak up as much liquid as possible, then apply the vinegar solution. If you're treating protein stains, such as baby formula, blood, cheese sauce, feces, milk, urine, and vomit, neutralize them by alternating this solution with ammonia. To treat ink stains, apply alcohol first, then glycerin, before using this solution.

½–4 tablespoons rosemary essential oil
1 cup vinegar
1 tablespoon liquid dishwashing detergent
½ cup water

1. Combine all the ingredients in a glass spray bottle.
2. Shake to combine. Because the oil and vinegar don't mix well, you'll need to continue shaking during use. Apply to the stain, and rub gently. Allow it to set for 15 minutes, then launder.
Storage. Label and store in a glass bottle; it keeps indefinitely.

Rosemary-Alcohol Stain Remover for Grass Stains

Use this stain remover on nonwashable fabrics. It may cause dyes to run, so use a pad beneath the stain when treating. You may have to treat the entire item with the solution to maintain even color.

½–4 tablespoons rosemary essential oil
1 cup alcohol (isopropyl or ethyl)

1. Combine the ingredients in a glass spray bottle.
2. With a pad beneath the stain, spray on, then blot with a clean, dry cloth. If color runs, soak the entire item in the solution. Allow it to dry in a ventilated area before having the piece dry-cleaned.

Storage. Store for up to 1 year in a labeled glass spray bottle.

Variation for Washables

For washable fabrics, add 2 tablespoons liquid detergent to the rosemary grass stain solution. Spray on stains, and then launder.

Rosemary-Alcohol Stain Remover for Grease

Although this stain remover is designed for use on washable fabrics, it may cause dyes to run, so use a pad beneath the stain when treating. You may have to submerge the entire item in the solution in order to maintain even color.

Fuller's earth
½–4 tablespoons rosemary essential oil
1 cup alcohol (isopropyl or ethyl)

1. Cover the grease stain with fuller's earth and allow it to set while you prepare alcohol solution.
2. Combine the essential oil and alcohol in a glass spray bottle.
3. Vacuum or shake off the fuller's earth, then, with a pad beneath the stain, spray the stain with the alcohol solution. Blot with a clean, dry cloth.

Storage. Store in a labeled glass spray bottle for up to 1 year.

Rosemary-Soap Stain Remover

Hand-washables like lingerie and nylons need gentle care, but they may also have picked up stubborn stains. Mix up a batch of this formula so that it's available for everything you hand-wash.

½–4 tablespoons rosemary essential oil
½–4 tablespoons glycerin
1 cup liquid castile soap
Herbal vinegar

1. Using equal amounts of essential oil and glycerin, combine the two in a small mixing bowl.
2. Pour the oil-glycerin mix into a glass bottle, add the castile soap, and blend thoroughly.
3. Dampen the article to be cleaned, and apply the soap solution directly to the stain. Rub gently. Wash the entire article in a dilute solution of the soap. Add a splash of herbal vinegar to the rinse water to remove soap residue.

Storage. Store in a labeled glass or plastic bottle for up to 6 months.

Rosemary-Peroxide Stain Pretreatment

A pretreatment for stains on silks and wools, this formula works especially hard on perspiration stains, and lightens white and cream-colored silks and wools. (Never use chlorine bleach on silk or wool; it damages and yellows them.) For perspiration stains on cotton, lay the garment in the sun all day, spraying it several times to keep it damp.

½ tablespoon rosemary essential oil
1 cup hydrogen peroxide

1. Combine the essential oil and peroxide in a glass spray bottle.
2. Shake well before and during use. Spray on stain until quite wet, and allow it to sit for ½ hour. After treatment, launder, adding herbal vinegar to the final rinse.

Storage. Hydrogen peroxide loses its potency within a month of being opened, so make only what you can use within that time.

Rosemary-Murphy's Stain Pretreatment

A good pretreatment for greasy stains on washable fabrics, this combination is also an excellent soap for washing goose-down pillows and comforters.

½–4 tablespoons rosemary essential oil
1 cup Murphy's Oil Soap

1. Combine the essential oil with Murphy's Oil Soap in a glass jar.
2. Apply to grease stains or combination stains on washable fabrics. Moisten fabric first, and work the mixture into the stain. Let it set for at least 15 minutes before washing, or overnight if the stain is old.

Storage. Store for 1 year in a labeled glass bottle.

Rosemary-Lifetree Stain Pretreatment

This pretreatment works well on many types of stains on washable fabrics. Remember to use cold water when you are treating stains, as hot water sets many stains and makes them harder to remove.

½–4 tablespoons rosemary essential oil
I cup Lifetree's Premium Dishwashing Liquid with Aloe and Calendula

1. Combine the essential oil with the dishwashing liquid in a glass spray bottle.
2. Apply to stains on dampened, washable fabrics. Scrub with a fingernail brush, if fabric is durable enough. Allow to set for 15 minutes, then launder.

Storage. Store in a labeled glass spray bottle; it keeps indefinitely.

Rosemary and Fuller's Earth Grease Remover

Use this mixture for treating grease stains on upholstery, rugs, woolen fabrics, fabrics with nap (like velvet), as well as unwashable textiles. Fuller's earth is available at hobby stores and home centers.

½–4 tablespoons rosemary essential oil
1 cup fuller's earth

1. Combine the essential oil and fuller's earth. Stir, or whirl in a blender to combine thoroughly.
2. Sprinkle the mixture onto the stain until it is fully covered. If you're cleaning a fabric with a nap, use a brush to gently work the mixture into the fibers. Allow it to set for at least 1 hour, or as long as overnight, until the grease is absorbed.
3. Vacuum, or gently dust off the mixture and discard. Repeat, if necessary.

Storage. Store in a labeled glass jar or metal container for one year.

Rosemary-Glycerin Stain Pretreatment

This is a useful pretreatment for greasy stains like butter, cooking oil, mayonnaise, or margarine on washable fabrics. See the variations below for other uses.

½–4 tablespoons rosemary essential oil
1 cup glycerin

1. Combine the essential oil and glycerin in a glass bottle.
2. Apply directly to stain and allow it to soak in. If necessary, follow the variation "for most other stains" below before laundering.

Storage. Store in a labelled glass bottle for a year or more.

Rosemary-Glycerin Variations

For coffee, tea, and other tannin stains on nonwashable fabrics, combine this solution with an equal amount of isopropyl alcohol. Before treating, test for color fastness on a seam. Place an absorbent pad beneath the stain. Apply the solution to the stain and blot gently. Repeat if necessary. Allow to dry in an area with good air circulation, then dryclean.

For most other stains, including combinations like coffee with cream, combine 1 tablespoon of the glycerin-essential oil solution with 1 tablespoon liquid dishwashing detergent and ½ cup water. Apply directly to the stain and leave on for 15 minutes, then wash the article.

LAUNDRY POWDERS AND PASTES

Essential oils add both wonderful fragrance and solvent properties to these useful laundry products. Try the powders as laundry boosters to lift dirt and grease, and mix them with water, liquid dish soap, or castile soap to make stain removal pastes for badly soiled items. Rosemary is my favorite essential oil for laundry products, but if you're pregnant, you should substitute lavender. Blends of rosemary and lavender essential oils appeal to both men and women, so they're a good compromise for the family laundry.

Rosemary and Color-Safe Bleach Presoak

Keep this formula on your laundry shelf for stains on washable colored fabrics, as well as white fabrics that you do not wish to bleach with liquid laundry bleach.

½–4 tablespoons rosemary essential oil
1 cup all-fabric bleach powder (sodium perborate)

1. Combine essential oil with bleach powder. Stir, or whirl in a blender to combine thoroughly.
2. Presoak stained fabrics in a solution containing ¼ cup of the rosemary-bleach mixture and 5 gallons of water for 1 hour. (For perspiration stains, soak overnight.) Launder, using ½–¾ cup of the rosemary-bleach mixture in the machine-wash load along with detergent.

Storage. Keeps for 6–12 months in a labeled glass jar or metal container, stored in a cool, dark place. Shake before use.

Rosemary-Baking Soda Laundry Powder

This powder goes to work to neutralize acid stains and absorb odor. If you prefer using a paste-style product (for stubborn stains or for articles that can't be laundered), add water, a few tablespoonsful at a time, to the powder mixture. Or, for an extra boost, use Lifetree's Dishwashing Liquid or another liquid detergent instead of water. Allow to dry, then remove the residue by brushing or vacuuming.

½–4 tablespoons rosemary essential oil
1 cup baking soda

1. Combine essential oil and baking soda by hand or in a blender.
2. Add ½ cup to a full washer load along with detergent.
Storage. Store in a labeled, covered glass jar or metal container; it keeps indefinitely.

Rosemary-Borax Laundry Powder

Borax works on mildew stains and neutralizes odors like urine. For difficult stains and unwashables, make a laundry paste by adding water or liquid detergent to the powder. Apply, allow to dry, then brush off the residue.

½–4 tablespoons essential oil
1 cup borax

1. Thoroughly combine essential oil and borax by hand or in a blender.
2. Add ½ cup to a full washer load along with laundry detergent.
Storage. Store in a labeled, covered glass jar or metal container; it keeps indefinitely.

Rosemary-Washing Soda Laundry Powder

This is the mixture to use for greasy dirt. If you have particularly stubborn stains or the article can't be laundered, make a laundry paste by gradually adding water or liquid detergent to the powder. Apply, allow to dry, then brush or vacuum off the residue.

½–4 tablespoons rosemary essential oil
1 cup washing soda

1. Combine essential oil and washing soda by hand or in a blender.
2. Add ½ cup to a full washer load along with detergent.
3. Add ¼ to 1 cup of herbal vinegar to the rinse water to prevent graying of whites and dulling of colors.
Storage. Store in a labeled, covered glass jar or metal container; it keeps indefinitely.

Leather Cleaners

Like all skins, leather requires frequent cleaning and moisturizing. These leather formulas can be used on the outside of suitcases, briefcases, shoes, handbags, and furniture. After cleaning your leather, condition with Leather Cream (page 122). Very dry, old leathers may need to be conditioned more than once.

Leather furniture will last longer if it is positioned away from the drying heat of direct sunlight, heating vents, radiators, or woodstoves. If that's not possible, keep a close eye on it, and if it seems to be losing its resiliency, wash and moisturize the leather more often.

Essential Oil-Enhanced Murphy's Oil Soap Concentrate for Leather

Wash leather with this solution to remove grease and grime. The stronger fragrances of roots, woods, and gums complement the scent of leather.

> 2 tablespoons of your favorite essential oil (see page 121 for suggestions)
> 1 cup Murphy's Oil Soap Concentrate (available in paint stores)
> ½ cup dried herbs (see page 121 for suggestions)
> 1½ cups water
> ¼ cup herbal vinegar
> 1 quart warm water

1. In a small bowl, stir the essential oil into the Murphy's. Beat well to disperse the oil completely.
2. Prepare an herbal infusion, using the dried herbs and 1½ cups of water. Allow to steep for 15 minutes, covered, to retain heat and fragrance. Strain into a large bowl.
3. Add 1 tablespoon of the essential oil-Murphy's mixture to the hot infusion. Whisk to a froth. Apply to leather with a sponge or soft cloth; for stiff leathers, you can use a natural bristle brush to scrub gently.

4. Rinse with a mixture of the herbal vinegar and warm water. Wipe dry with a clean cloth.

Storage. Keep the concentrated soap in a cool dark place in a labeled glass jar or metal container for up to 6 months.

PERSONAL FAVORITE

For 4 cups Murphy's Oil Soap Concentrate, use 5 tablespoons lavender essential oil, 2 tablespoons orange essential oil, and 1 tablespoon rosemary essential oil. *For the herbal infusion,* use calamus, cedarwood, rosewood, sandalwood, clary sage, patchouli, and/or lavender.

Lanolin and Murphy's Leather Treatment

Leathers need to be moisturized as well as cleaned. This formula treats dry, cracked leathers that have been badly treated, neglected, and/or improperly stored at high temperatures when wet. Lanolin is quite sticky; use the larger amount only if the leather is very dry and cracked.

> 2 tablespoons essential oil (such as lavender, orange, or rosemary)
> 1 cup Murphy's Oil Soap Concentrate
> 1–3 tablespoons lanolin

1. Combine the essential oil with the Murphy's Soap Concentrate.

2. Stir in the lanolin with a heavy spoon. The mixture will look exactly like whipped butter.

3. Rub soap mixture directly into the leather. Allow it to set for a few minutes up to an hour, while the leather softens. Work in further with your fingers or a soft brush.

4. Blend 1 tablespoon of the soap mixture with 1 quart of hot water, cool slightly, then rinse the leather.

5. If the leather is extremely dry, repeat the process, but leave the undiluted soap on the leather overnight to absorb more lanolin. Rinse with a fresh diluted soap solution, as in step 4, followed by a rinse containing ¼ cup vinegar in 1 quart of water.

Storage. Store the concentrated soap in a labeled glass jar or metal container in a cool, dark place for up to 6 months.

Leather Cream

Making leather cream is a two-part process. It's very important to get both solutions to the right temperature at the same time. If the infusion is too cold, some of the wax will precipitate out, forming gritty bits, and the emulsion won't whip up properly.

½ cup dried herbs (or 1 cup fresh)
    (see page 123 for suggestions)
1½ cups water
    1 cup plain or herb-infused walnut, olive, mineral, or jojoba oil
    1 tablespoon essential oil (see page 123 for suggestions)
    1 ounce cocoa butter
    ¾ ounce beeswax

1. Place the herbs in a heat-proof container.
2. Boil water. Pour boiling water over herbs, and stir to combine. Cover. Allow to steep while you proceed to the next step.
3. Combine the oil with the cocoa butter and beeswax in the double boiler. Heat over low to medium heat until the wax is melted. Remove from heat. Allow to cool just until a crescent of wax forms at the edge of the pan.
4. Strain 1 cup plus 1 tablespoon of the infusion into a measuring cup. The temperature should be 95° to 105°F. If it's too cool, warm the infusion in a microwave oven; if it's too hot, allow it to cool. (Return the oil solution to heat so it doesn't skim over completely.)

5. Pour the infusion into a blender. With the lid on, turn the blender on high, and quickly pour in the oil solution, using a funnel if necessary to direct the solution in through the access opening in the lid. Allow the blender to run continuously while the emulsion forms. If the solution is a little too hot, it may take 5 minutes or a little longer.
6. Once the mixture has thickened, turn off the blender and scrape down the sides with a spatula. Allow it to cool for at least 15 minutes.
7. Add up to 1 tablespoon of the essential oil and blend again.

Use. Rub leather cream into leather with a soft cloth. Allow the mixture to be absorbed into the leather for at least 24 hours, then burnish dry with a soft cloth.

Storage. Label and cover, then store in the refrigerator or freezer to prevent rancidity or fungi from forming. Keeps for about 6 months.

PERSONAL FAVORITES
Herb-infused oil: Calendula and chamomile flowers
Essential oils: Sandalwood (preferred), vetiver, patchouli, cedarwood, clary sage, or rosewood

AIR FRESHENERS AND SWEETENERS

Nothing smells better than clean, fresh air. Here are some first-aid solutions for refreshing stale air that bring garden fragrances indoors and put them to work for you.

Vinegar Bowl

A shallow bowl containing vinegar, set out overnight in a room, is a simple, but tried-and-true method for banishing damp, musty, or smoky odors. For a fragrant herbal twist, use sweet-scented herbal vinegars, like rose, anise hyssop, sweet woodruff, or sweet grass, or raspberry vinegar and sweet grass. You can make a one-herb vinegar, called a "simple," or an herb combination. Include a fixative like sweet grass or sweet woodruff to extend the solution's life.

You can strain the solution or leave interesting fruits and flowers or sweet grass braids (see pages 133–134) in the bowl. Choose a decorative, preferably flat-bottomed, shallow glass storage bowl that holds about 2 quarts of water, with a tight-fitting lid, so the solution can be used again and again.

lid

Float flowers and pieces of braid in the vinegar solution.

Safety first. Don't leave the vinegar solution where small children or pets can spill it or drink from it.

> 7 cups dried herbs or 11 cups fresh herbs
> (see below for suggestions)
> 1 gallon distilled white, cider, or other fruit-flavored vinegar
> 1 cup sweet grass or sweet woodruff, as a fixative
> 1 tablespoon allspice, cinnamon, cloves, or ginger

1. Place the herbs in a gallon jar, and pour the vinegar over them, filling the jar with liquid. Be sure all herbs are covered completely. Cover the jar. Allow to infuse for at least a week.

2. Strain, if you wish. Decant most of the vinegar into display bowl.

Use. Set the vinegar bowl on a stable surface and remove the lid. As vinegar evaporates from the bowl, add more from the storage container. Cover the bowl when its effects are not needed.

Storage. The strained vinegar lasts for several years if kept in a glass jar in a cool, dark place. If unstrained, remove any plant material that is exposed to air when the level of the liquid drops.

PERSONAL FAVORITES

Principal herb: Anise hyssop, citrus peels, costmary, eucalyptus, frankincense, fruit-scented sage, jasmine, juniper berries, lavender, lemon mint, meadowsweet, orangemint, rosemary, roses, spearmint, sweet Annie, sweet grass, sweet woodruff, or Thuja cedar leaf

Additional herbs: Chamomile, heather, lemon balm, lemon verbena, lemongrass, linden flowers, pineapple sage, or sweet Cicely

Fresh Herbal Spray

This light, refreshing spray is healthful and inexpensive to make. If you use fresh herbs, double the quantities suggested. A fixative will help the fragrance linger; try angelica or calamus root, cedarwood, oakmoss, sandalwood, sweet grass, or sweet woodruff. Avoid gummy or resinous fixatives like copal, frankincense, and myrrh, which can clog the sprayer mechanism. Calculate the amount of fixative as part of the total ½ cup of herbs. This recipe makes about ¾ cup, enough to freshen the whole house a couple of times.

Safety first. Be careful not to get spray into eyes.

> ½ cup dried herbs (see below for suggestions)
> 1 cup water
> 1 or more tablespoons fixative (optional)

1. Place herbs in heat-proof container. Boil water and pour it over the herbs; stir rapidly. Cover the container and allow to steep until cool (at least ½ hour).
2. Strain. If you see bits of plant material that could clog the spray mechanism, strain again through a water-dampened paper coffee filter. Pour into a spray bottle, using a funnel if necessary.

Use. Spray into the air all around the house.

Storage. This will keep in the refrigerator for a few days.

PERSONAL FAVORITES

Lavender herb: 6 tablespoons dried lavender, 2 tablespoons dried rosemary, 10 bay leaves

Sweet rose: 6 tablespoons dried rosebuds, 2 tablespoons dried sweet woodruff

Candy-scented: 4 tablespoons dried anise hyssop, 2 tablespoons dried chamomile, 2 tablespoons dried sweet Annie, ½ teaspoon whole allspice

Light mint: 2 tablespoons dried lemon balm, 2 tablespoons dried lemon peel, 2 tablespoons dried spearmint, 2 tablespoons dried Thuja cedar leaves

Disinfectant Spray

Both the alcohol and essential oils in this herbal infusion kills microorganisms in the air and on surfaces. The more essential oil you use, the more powerful the disinfectant. I prefer to use 190-proof potable ethyl alcohol. Isopropyl alcohol is also effective, and less expensive, but its strong odor competes with the herbs. You can also use vodka, gin, or light rum.

Safety first. When made with isopropyl or denatured alcohol, this solution is toxic if ingested. Do not spray into eyes. Avoid spraying on shellacked and varnished wood surfaces, as alcohol and essential oils may mar them.

> ½ cup dried herbs (see below for suggestions)
> 1 cup water
> ½ cup alcohol
> 1–2 teaspoons essential oil (see page 127 for suggestions)

1. Make an infusion with the herbs and water, and allow to steep until cool (at least ½ hour).
2. Strain. If you see bits of plant material that could clog the spray mechanism, strain again through a water-dampened paper coffee filter. Measure out ½ cup, and set aside.
3. Place alcohol in a glass spray bottle; add the essential oils. Pour in the reserved herb infusion. Shake well.

Use. Spray into the air all around the house.

Storage. Label carefully. Keeps for six months — longer, if refrigerated.

Bathroom Disinfectant Spray

For a bathroom spray, measure 1 cup isopropyl alcohol into a spray bottle. Add 2½ teaspoons eucalyptus, fir, lavender, lemon, lemon eucalyptus, orange, peppermint, pine, rosemary, spearmint, spruce, tea tree, or white thyme essential oil. Make up more than one kind and vary the usage from week to week, so that microorganisms don't develop resistance to your mixture.

Lavender Lover: ½ cup dried lavender for the infusion; 1 to 2 teaspoons lavender essential oil

Lemon Eucalyptus: ½ cup dried eucalyptus for the infusion; 1 teaspoon lemon essential oil and 1 teaspoon lemon eucalyptus essential oil

Antiseptic Rose: ¼ cup dried roses and ¼ cup dried hyssop for the infusion; 1 teaspoon rose geranium essential oil and 1 teaspoon rosewood essential oil

Sweet Orange: 3 tablespoons each of dried anise hyssop, sweet Annie, and thyme for the infusion; 1 to 2 teaspoons orange essential oil

Beeswax Pastilles

Handy for scenting drawers and closets, pastilles are made of melted beeswax scented with essential oils that is poured into small molds. When the scent evaporates, you can melt and recast them, adding more essential oil. This recipe makes 18 large, or about 36 small, pastilles.

Safety first. Wax is flammable, so always use a double boiler and avoid open flames. These are strongly scented, so work with a window open or an exhaust fan on. Keep pastilles out of the reach of small children.

Mineral or jojoba oil, for oiling the molds

4 ounces yellow beeswax

2–3 tablespoons essential oil (see page 128)

Beeswax pastilles shaped as acorns

1. Lightly oil the molds with mineral or jojoba oil.
2. Place the beeswax in double boiler and melt it over low heat. Remove from heat and allow it to cool just until wax begins to solidify at the edge of the pan.
3. Quickly add the essential oils, stir well, and ladle the mixture into the molds.
4. Allow to cool, then pop the pastilles out of the molds and place them oiled-side-down on paper towels. Pat gently to absorb oil. Seal matching pastilles back to back while the wax is still slightly warm and sticky, if you'd like.

PERSONAL FAVORITES

Lemon Candy: 1 tablespoon plus 1 teaspoon lemon essential oil, 2 teaspoons tangerine essential oil, 2 teaspoons balsam of Peru

Sweet Lavender: 1 tablespoon plus 1 teaspoon lavender essential oil, 2 teaspoons rosemary essential oil, 2 teaspoons tangerine essential oil, 1 teaspoon frankincense

Moth Chaser: 1 tablespoon lavandin essential oil, 2 teaspoons rosemary essential oil, 1 teaspoon white camphor oil, 1 teaspoon cedarwood essential oil

Pantry Pastilles: For kitchen cabinets, use bug-chasing essential oils like bay leaf, black pepper, cedarwood, citrus fruits, lavandin, rosemary, sage, spike lavender, white camphor, or yarrow.

Easy Wax Cleanup

To clean up, reheat the double boiler and the ladle until the remnants of the wax melt, then wipe the pan out with a paper towel. For stubborn residue, use turpentine, then wash with hot soapy water. (Reserve a double boiler for housekeeping preparations, and do not use the same one for cooking.)

Moth-Away Sachets

Many herbs are moth-chasers, but unfortunately, their scents are sometimes not much more appealing to us than they are to the moths. This combination smells pretty good and keeps its fragrance for a long time because it contains six fixatives.

> 2 cups each cedarwood and dried wormwood
> 1½ cups each dried lavender and dried tansy
> ¼ cup dried sweet woodruff
> 1 cup oakmoss
> ½ cup each dried patchouli, sandalwood, dried southernwood, vetiver root, dried rosemary, whole cloves

1. Powder all ingredients by whirling them in a coffee grinder or spice mill. Mix well.
2. Age for 2 to 4 weeks in a glass jar, then make up sachets.

Simple Sachet Bag

For a 3-inch-square sachet, cut a piece of fabric 4" x 9". Fold the fabric in half crosswise, right sides together. Sew both side seams, taking a ½-inch seam allowance (A). Turn the raw edge under ¼ inch, and then turn under again; stitch along the fold. Turn the bag right side out. Fill about two-thirds full with sachet (B).

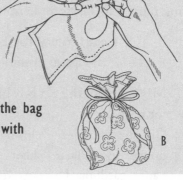

Shoe Bag Sachets

This formula covers up odors that emanate from stinky sneakers. For especially bad problems, use zeolite or baking soda in shoes while waiting for the fragrance blend to age. (Baking soda makes leather brittle, so it's best to keep its use to a minimum.)

> 3 cups natural clay cat box litter
> 3–9 tablespoons essential oil (see below for suggestions)

Mix together the cat box litter and oil. Age in a glass jar for a week. **Use.** Fill socks or pantyhose with the scented clay pellets. Close off the ends with rubber bands. Cover the rubber bands with a ribbon or a bit of twine, if you wish. Place in shoes and leave overnight or longer.

PERSONAL FAVORITES

Sweet Mix: Equal parts orange and balsam of Peru essential oils, with a touch of lemon essential oil

Icy Winter Winds: 1 tablespoon peppermint essential oil, 1 teaspoon rosemary essential oil, ½ teaspoon clove essential oil, ½ teaspoon patchouli essential oil, ¼ teaspoon white camphor essential oil (do not use this combination if you are pregnant)

Scented Drawer Liners

If you use fancy papers, these liners will make a lovely gift. You don't need to discard the cat box litter pellets after use: Refresh them with additional essential oil and reuse them to make sachets or for scenting more papers; store them in a sealed glass jar.

1 quart natural clay cat box litter
4–12 tablespoons essential oil (your favorite)

1. Mix together the cat box litter and oil. Age in a glass jar for a week.
2. Cut sheets of drawer lining paper to drawer size. Place a sheet of heavy paper, cardboard, or waxed paper, also cut to size, on the top and bottom of the lining paper pile. Roll the entire pile into a loose cylinder. If the paper is printed on one side, roll that side to the outside. Bind the cylinder with string.

Roll drawer paper and cardboard loosely together.

3. Line a box that is large enough to hold the cylinder with aluminum foil to seal in the fragrance.
4. Place the cat box litter mix in the container with the paper cylinder, carefully tucking the pellets under, inside, and on top of the roll, so as not to crush the paper. Cover the container, and seal it with tape. Leave in a cool, dry place for a month.

Use. Remove the litter, shake or brush off any dust, and unroll the paper. Place the papers in drawers.

Sweet Bags

These old-fashioned, large, flat sachets will line the shelves of your linen closet, permeating linens with sweet fragrances and also chasing away any unwanted pests. The amounts given here are enough to fill one 12 by 36-inch sweet bag. You will need tightly woven cotton fabric, such as an old sheet, to make the bag.

10 cups each of dried and crumbled costmary leaves, lavender
flowers, and sweet woodruff leaves

1–2 tablespoons lavender essential oil

3 cups calamus root, chopped small before drying, or purchased
cut and sifted

1. Combine the herbs, essential oil, and calamus root in a glass jar, cover, and allow to age in a cool, dark place for several weeks.

2. Measure your shelves, and for each shelf, cut two fabric pieces 1 inch bigger than the shelves all around. With right sides of the fabric facing, stitch along three sides and part of the fourth, taking up a 1-inch seam allowance. Leave a 6-inch opening. Turn the piece right side out, and fill with the herb mixture. Stitch the opening closed.

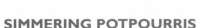

Fill the prepared bag loosely with herb mix.

SIMMERING POTPOURRIS

My favorite way to spread the joys of herbal scents throughout our home is by simmering our favorite botanicals. I keep a large pot of potpourri mixture simmering on the back burner of the stove most of the winter, and the fine vapor adds moisture to our dry, heated air while it disseminates fragrances that not only lift our spirits, but also invisibly battle airborne microbes.

If you have favorite dry potpourri mixes loaded with woods, barks, roots, and spices, you may be able to simmer them, although the ratios of the ingredients may have to be changed. For instance, the fragrance of dried thyme intensifies when simmered, even over-coming the usually strong, spicy aroma of cloves. Mints, lemon balm, and lemon verbena have ephemeral fragrances that must be replenished frequently. Citrus fruit peels are wonderful, but when their essential oils evaporate, they simply smell like cooked fruit.

Aromatic Air Cleanser Simmering Potpourri

Unlike dried potpourri, simmering potpourri does not need a fixative to blend its scents and make them last longer. Here, however, the fixative calamus adds its own unique fragrance.

> 2 cups dried Thuja cedar leaves (arborvitae) and twigs
>
> 1 cup each calamus root, elecampane root, and flowering hyssop tops

Combine all ingredients and mix well.

Use. Use about 1 cup in 4 cups of water, and simmer until the fragrance is gone.

Storage. Store remaining dry mixture in a glass jar in a cool, dark place.

All-American Simmering Potpourri

For a uniquely American brew, use only native plants, including deer's tongue *(Trilisa odoratissima)*, fruit-scented sage *(Salvia dorisiana)*, and linden *(Tilia americana)*.

> 2 cups each deer's tongue leaves, anise hyssop, fruit-scented sage, and linden flowers
>
> 20"–24" sweet grass braid (see page 133)

Combine all ingredients and mix well.

Use. Use about 1 cup of the mixture and about 2 inches of sweet grass braid in 4 cups of water. Simmer until the fragrance is exhausted.

Storage. Store the dry mixture in a glass jar in a cool, dark place.

Potpourri for Pennies

- Take advantage of seasonal sales and store markdowns on citrus fruits. Dry or freeze any you don't use immediately.
- Collect small fruits, rosehips, and orchard deadfalls. Use garden and houseplant prunings and pinchings, including fragrant twigs, barks, leaves, buds, flowers, and seeds.
- Use up spices and dried herbs that have outlived their culinary usefulness.

Sinus-Clearing Simmer

Developed as a steam to help clear up bronchial problems, this formula can double as a facial steaming blend if you have oily or troubled skin. You can also infuse it in vinegar for use in cleaning.

> 4 cups dried lavender
>
> 3 cups dried eucalyptus leaves
>
> 1 cup each bay leaves, dried grapefruit peel, dried lemon peel, dried rosemary, dried roses, and dried sage
>
> ½ cup each cinnamon chips, whole allspice, and whole cloves
>
> 2 tablespoons, plus 1½ teaspoons each whole black peppercorns and whole cardamom pods

Combine all ingredients and toss to mix thoroughly.

Use. Use about 1 cup at a time in 4 cups of simmering water. Add more water and/or herb mix, as needed. When the fragrance is finally exhausted, toss the residue into the compost.

Storage. Store dry mixture in a glass jar in a cool, dark place.

Sweet Grass Braids

Dried sweet grass has a distinctive sweet aroma, similar to newly mown hay. The braided dry grass is used in decorations, in simmering potpourris, or as incense. If you have enough sweet grass, make a number of braids the same length, then bind the ends together with ribbons or twine to make a garland. To use as incense, a traditional Native American custom, carefully light the end of the braid. When it is lit, blow out the flame and allow it to smolder. Re-apply flame if needed to keep the braid smoldering. The aroma is a bit like that of burning autumn leaves, only sweeter. If you plan to burn the braid, use grass for the fastening and don't braid ribbon into the strands.

1. Harvest sweet grass stems by cutting an inch above the base. Gather a bundle of about 3 dozen stems of grass. Hold the bundle in your hand as you cut, keeping the stem ends facing in the same direction. Don't pick stems with flower or seed spikes.

2. Rubberband each bundle immediately after gathering, and hang it to dry until the sweet haylike scent develops.

3. Combine the stems into bundles each about 1 inch in diameter, and fasten them together again with a rubberband. Dip the bundle into warm water to give it some flexibility and then (leaving the rubberband in place) divide it into three equal parts.

4. Use the traditional braiding method, alternating right side over center, left side over center until the braid is done. For a fancier braid, incorporate narrow colored ribbons in with the strands as you braid. Rubberband the finished end and hang it up to dry.

Braid a bundle of sweetgrass.

5. Replace the rubberband with a wrapping of sweet grass, natural twine, or dyed raffia.

Lavender Bundles

Because I'm sometimes too impatient to weave lavender wands, I invented this easier version. Harvest prime lavender in bloom and in bud.

1. Bundle together any reasonable number of lavender stems, from 15 to 25, even or odd. Cut the stems to about 8 inches. Rubberband them under the flower heads.

2. Bend the stems over the flower heads, starting about 1 inch beneath the rubberband. Fold the stems neatly over the flower heads, caging them nicely, and spreading the stems evenly. Fasten with a rubberband, and trim stems, leaving about 1 inch beyond the rubberband.

3. Dry the bundle on a rack for 1 or 2 weeks.

4. Cover the rubberband by wrapping it with a colorful ⅜-inch-wide ribbon tied in a bow.

Sleep Pillow Blend

Now that your home is sparkling and smells fantastic, you've earned a night of calm, sweet sleep and wonderful dreams. This dried herb combination makes a pleasant, slightly sweet aromatic fragrance with a calming effect. Relax and enjoy!

4½ cups sweet woodruff leaves

2 cups lavender flowers

1¾ cups rose petals

1 cup each of chamomile flowers, jasmine flowers, and oakmoss lichen

½ cup each of angelica root chips, calamus root chips or slices, and linden flowers

4 tablespoons each of meadowsweet, mugwort leaves, and yarrow flowers

2 tablespoons each of anise seed and yellow sandalwood chips

1. Combine all of the dried herbs until well blended, crushing the leaves gently between your fingers to break them up into smaller bits, and place the mixture in a large, covered glass jar.

2. Age the blend in a cool, dark place for 4 weeks, then stuff the herbs into a zippered neckroll pillow case and cover with a heavy quilted case. Tuck this pillow in among your bed pillows or under your neck before you go to sleep each night.

YOUR HERBAL CLEANING CLOSET

On the following pages are several invaluable charts with information about the ingredients used in many of the housekeeping formulas in the book. Herbal Housekeeping Ingredients describes the many useful additives and bases that are included in the recipes. In addition to information about the appearance and characteristics of each ingredient, the chart tells you how to use it most effectively and where you can purchase it. This is followed by charts listing fixatives and essential oils that enhance and strengthen your cleaning products. We hope you'll find these references handy as you explore this new world of sweet-smelling, effective herbal housekeeping.

NAME	WHERE TO PURCHASE	PHYSICAL APPEARANCE
Baking soda (sodium bicarbonate)	Grocery store (Arm and Hammer)	Soft, white crystalline powder
Beeswax	Local beekeeper (for best price)	Soft, honey-scented wax produced by bees; naturally golden in color, but bleached for cosmetic products
Bentonite (sodium bentonite)	White to grayish white powder	Clay, formed by the decomposition of volcanic ash
Borax (sodium tetraborate decahydrate)	Grocery store (Mule Team)	White powdery mineral
Boric acid	Pharmacy, home center, hardware store (in the pesticide department)	Odorless white powder, created by adding sulfuric or hydrochloric acid to borax solution
Bran	Health food store	Outer, fibrous coating of cereal grains
Carnauba wax	Woodworking supplier	Very hard wax derived from the leaves of the Brazilian wax palm tree
Castile bar and liquid soaps	Health food store, mail-order supplier (Dr. Bronner's Liquid Castile and Bar Soaps, Kiss My Face, Baby Liquid Castile)	Bar or liquid soap
Chalk (calcium carbonate)	Grocery store (Bon Ami)	White powdery mineral derived from limestone
Citric acid	Grocery store, mail-order supplier	White crystalline powder made from lemon, lime, or pineapple juice by mold fermentation
Citrus solvent	Health food store, mail-order supplier (Citra-Solv)	Translucent orange liquid
Clay-based cat box litter	Grocery store, pet supply store	Absorbent clay pellets
Cocoa butter	Health food store, pharmacy, mail-order supplier	Fatty substance, solid at room temperature, extracted from cacao beans
Cream of tartar	Grocery store, mail-order supplier	White crystalline powder, a by-product of winemaking
Diatomaceous earth	Garden supply store, swimming pool supplier (Concern)	Powder; the pulverized fossils of small ancient sea plants called diatoms
Fuller's earth	Ceramic or hobby store, home center	Porous clay

CHARACTERISTICS	USES
Abrasive, absorbent, acid neutralizer	Scouring powder, odor neutralizer, stain and spill absorber
Soluble in oils, but not in water, vinegar, glycerin, or alcohol; melting point is about 145°F; flammable	Wax, polish, candles, molds
Not soluble in water, but can absorb several times its volume in liquids	Stain and spill absorber
Soluble in water; moderately toxic	Cleaning and laundry products, insect pest control (microcrystalline residue harms roaches and other crawling insects)
Soluble in water, glycerin, and alcohol	Insect pest control (toxic to roaches)
Keeps well, as it lacks oils; oat bran is lighter in color than wheat bran, so residue shows less	Upholstery spot cleaner
Melting point 185°F; flammable (use double boiler to melt); may cause allergic reaction	Floor wax, furniture polish
Mild, unscented	Laundry detergent, surface cleaner
Only slightly soluble in water, but very soluble in acid solutions; mildly abrasive	Soft scrubber, metal polish
Antioxidant so it serves as a preservative; removes soap scum and mineral deposits	Preservative in many products; scouring powder
Made from citrus, augmented with essential and other oils, and a detergent	Thinner
Unscented	Sachets and other scented products
Pleasant, sweet, light-chocolate scent; melting point of about 92°F	Furniture cream, leather cream
Water-soluble leavening agent	Toilet cleaner, aluminum cleaner, spot remover
Gritty	Household and garden insect pest control
Highly absorptive	Grease remover

NAME	WHERE TO PURCHASE	PHYSICAL APPEARANCE
Herbal shampoo	Health food store, mail-order supplier	Liquid
Hydrogen peroxide	Pharmacy, health food store	Clear liquid
Incense charcoals	Religious goods store, mail-order supplier	Small, self-lighting briquettes of carbonized plant material
Jeweler's rouge (iron oxide)	Jewelry, hobby, or craft supply store	Fine reddish brown powder
Jojoba oil	Health food store, mail-order supplier	Wax derived from the seeds of a North American shrub (Simmondsia californica); looks like an oil
Lanolin	Pharmacy, mail-order supplier	Refined wool grease; light brown in color
Lifetree's Premium Dishwashing Liquid with Aloe & Calendula	Health food store, mail-order supplier	Liquid detergent
Mineral oil (liquid petrolatum)	Pharmacy	Clear oil distilled from petroleum
Mineral spirits	Paint store, home center	Clear liquid distilled from petroleum
Murphy's Oil Soap	Paint store	Vegetable-based soap made from pine bark; buy the jellylike concentrate
Paraffin wax	Craft or hobby supply store, hardware or grocery store	White wax derived from petroleum
Salt (sodium chloride)	Grocery or health food store (buy noniodized, pickling salt)	White, abrasive crystalline powder
Sodium perborate	Grocery store (as an "all-fabric bleach"), health food store	Odorless white powder
Turpentine	Paint or artist's supply store	Clear, volatile liquid with an oily feel, steam-distilled from the sap of trees (such as the longleaf pine and terebinth)
Vermiculite	Garden center	White, highly porous mineral
Washing soda, or soda ash	Grocery store	White powder
Zeolite	Dasun Company (see page 146)	Naturally occurring mineral found at the sites of active volcanoes

CHARACTERISTICS	USES
Sudsing liquid dissolves dirt and grease	Laundry agent for wool, cashmere, silk, goose down, and other animal fibers
Highly toxic in concentrated form, but available commercially in a 3% solution	Disinfectant; bleach for fabrics of protein origin, such as silk and wool
Used to burn gums, resins, or materials like sweet grass, which must remain in touch with a smoldering source of flame to burn	Incense
Soluble in acids	Metal polish
Does not go rancid	Wax, polish, wood finish
Strong odor	Leather restorer
Sudsing liquid dissolves dirt and grease	Stain pretreatment, hand-washing laundry product
Does not go rancid	Wax, polish, wood finish
Flammable	Paint thinner, floor wax
Pleasant fragrance	Surface cleaner, especially for painted and varnished wood
Soluble in turpentine, warm alcohol, and olive oil; melting point of about 140°F; flammable (use a double boiler to melt); less expensive than beeswax	Often mixed with beeswax in formulas and candles
Water soluble	Scouring powder
A natural bleach, releases oxygen when it decomposes in water	Bleach, disinfectant
Fresh, pungent, in-your-face aroma	Wood finish, floor and furniture wax, oil paint thinner
Insoluble except in hot acids	Container soil mixture
Soluble in water but not in alcohol; wear rubber gloves as it can irritate skin; moderately toxic	Laundry aid, surface cleaner, disinfectant
Has a negative charge (constantly attracts ions); can be solarized and used again	Odor and pollutant absorbant

Essential Oils for Housekeeping

ESSENTIAL OIL	CHARACTERISTICS AND USES	SAFETY LEVEL	PRICE
Anise	Sweet scent; relaxes and calms; promotes sleep; alleviates stress; disinfects	Safe to 2.5% dilution; higher dilution may cause skin irritation.	$$
Camphor, white	Repels insects and prevents hatching of larvae; counters depression	Least toxic of various forms of camphor; nonirritating and non-sensitizing; can cause convulsions; should be avoided by pregnant women and epileptics not on medication.	$
Cedarwood, red	Antiseptic; repels moths and insects; fixative	Nonirritating to skin.	$$
Cinnamon leaf	Warm, spicy fragrance, more medicinal than edible; cleans and disinfects	Safe to 10% dilution.	$$
Citronella	Repels mosquitoes	The citronellal it contains may be mildly irritating to the skin.	$
Clove bud	Antibacterial, antiparasitical, and antifungal; stimulates, energizes, and warms	Wear gloves and use it in low dilutions, as it can irritate the skin. Undiluted clove bud oil is strong enough to melt some plastics and to damage the surface of some metals, so use even diluted clove bud oil with caution, and test on a small area first.	$$$
Eucalyptus	Antibacterial (effective against staph, strep, pneumonia, and viruses); a 2 percent dilution, sprayed into the air, will kill 70 percent of airborne staph; antifungal	Nonirritating to skin.	$$
Fir	Pinelike fragrance; energizes, focuses, and uplifts	Use oil within 6 months to avoid skin irritation.	$$
Grapefruit	Citrus scent; stimulates pain relief (thus good for cleaning sickrooms)	Makes skin slightly sensitive to sunlight, so wear gloves. Avoid exposure to sun if 4% solution gets on skin.	$$

Key: $ = about $10–15 for 4 ounces
$$ = about $15–20 for 4 ounces
$$$ = about $20–25 for 4 ounces

Essential Oils for Housekeeping (continued)

ESSENTIAL OIL	CHARACTERISTICS AND USES	SAFETY LEVEL	PRICE
Lavender	Antibacterial, antiviral, and antifungal; calms, enhances immune system	Very safe.	$$$
Lemon	Antiviral and antibacterial (including staph, strep, and pneumonia); fresh, clean scent soothes and uplifts; negative charge attracts dust	Wear gloves. If dilution higher than 2% gets on skin, avoid sunlight for 12 hours.	$
Lemongrass	Disinfects; soothes; may protect against scabies and ringworm	Nonirritating, except to damaged skin.	$$
Lime	Refreshes, energizes, and uplifts	Causes skin to be sensitive to sun. Wear gloves. If dilution higher than 0.7% gets on skin, avoid sunlight for 12 hours.	$$
Orange, sweet	Antiviral, antibacterial, and antidepressant; enhances immune system; repels fleas	Very safe. Does not cause skin sensitivity to sun.	$
Peppermint	Antiviral, antiparasitical, and antibacterial; stimulates and energizes	Avoid exposure if you suffer from cardiac fibrillation.	$$
Pine	Antibacterial and antiviral; invigorates, energizes, and uplifts; stimulates immune system	Use within 6 months to avoid skin irritation.	$$
Rosemary	Antibacterial; activates the brain, memory, and energy; dissolves grease; repels insects (high camphor content)	Pregnant women and epileptics not on medication should avoid rosemary oil.	$$$
Rosewood	Antibacterial; rose geranium fragrance; induces tranquillity	Very safe.	$$$
Spearmint	Antidepressant, antiseptic	Safer than peppermint, since it lacks menthol and pulegone.	$$
Tangerine	Antiviral, antibacterial, and antidepressant; enhances immune system; repels fleas	Very safe.	$
Tea tree	Antibacterial, antiviral, antifungal, and antiseptic; enhances immune system	Very safe.	$$$

Fixatives for Housekeeping

COMMON NAME	BOTANICAL NAME	FORMS USED
Ambrette, Musk	*Hibiscus abelmoschus, H. moscheutos*	Seed, essential oil
Angelica	*Angelica archangelica*	Root, essential oil
Balsam of Peru	*Myroxylon pereirae*	Essential oil
Balsam of tolu	*Myroxylon balsamum*	Essential oil
Benzoin	*Styrax* species (especially *S. benzoin*)	Gum (powdered), absolute
Calamus	*Acorus americanus*	Root
Cedarwood	*Juniperus virginiana*	Wood chips, essential oil
Clary sage	*Salvia sclarea*	Flowers, buds, leaves, essential oil
Copaiba balsam	*Copaifera langsdorffii* (syn. *Copaiba officinalis*)	Gum
Copal, Amber	*Buresera fugaroides*	Gum
Deer's tongue	*Trilisa odoratissima*	Leaves
Frankincense	*Boswellia carterii*	Gum, in "tears" (droplets) or powdered, absolute
Galbanum	*Ferula galbaniflua*	Resin
Myrrh	*Commiphora myrrha*	Resin, absolute
Oakmoss lichen	*Evernia prunastri*	Lichen (whole or powdered), absolute

CHARACTERISTICS AND USES

SAFETY TIPS

CHARACTERISTICS AND USES	SAFETY TIPS
Sweet, sensual, earthy musklike scent	Essential oil is very safe for housekeeping uses.
Use with fruity, sweet, herbal, or woody fragrances	The essential oil causes phototoxic reactions (sunburn and blotchy skin).
Extremely sweet, vanilla-like fragrance; blends nicely with citrus fragrances; useful for taking the bitter, drying edge off other scents	May be a skin irritant.
Similar to balsam of Peru; combined with oil and used to treat raw wood, makes a hard, deliciously scented finish	May be a skin irritant.
Pleasantly scented white gum; use the powder in floral sachets; use the absolute in other fragrance products	May be a skin irritant; don't use the toxic tincture of benzoin (a different product altogether) as a fixative.
Aromatic, calming, somewhat medicinal fragrance	Essential oil is potentially carcinogenic.
Mellows with age; low, deep, grounding fragrance	Safe for housekeeping uses.
Relaxing, musklike, sweaty fragrance that improves with age	Essential oil contains estrogen-like substances, and should be avoided by those with breast cysts or cancer.
Fragrance similar to myrrh; oil used in soaps and perfumes	Safe for housekeeping uses.
Pleasant, though not as sweet or strong as frankincense; can be burned as an incense or fumigant	Safe for housekeeping uses.
Strongly sweet and somewhat fruity scent	Safe for housekeeping uses.
Sweet, uplifting, powerful but not coercive; burn as incense or incorporate the tears or powdered gum into sachets, and potpourris	Safe for housekeeping uses.
Sharp, strong, green, woody, somewhat spicy aroma	Safe for housekeeping uses.
Pungent and aromatic; burn as incense, incorporate in sachets and potpourris; extract resin in alcohol	Safe for housekeeping uses.
Sweet fragrance; blends well with woody or haylike scents (such as sweet woodruff); insect repellent	May cause skin irritation; contains toxic thujones; avoid during pregnancy.

COMMON NAME	BOTANICAL NAME	FORMS USED
Orrisroot	*Iris germanica* var. *florentina*	Root, absolute
Patchouli	*Pogostemon cablin*	Leaves, essential oil
Queen Anne's lace	*Daucus carota*	Seed, essential oil (sold as "carrot seed oil")
Red sandalwood	*Pterocarpus santalinus*	Wood
Storax	*Styrax officinalis*	Resin
Sweet clover, Melilot	*Melilotus officinalis*	Flowers, buds, leaves
Sweet grass	*Hierochloe odorata*	Grass blades
Sweet woodruff	*Galium odoratum*	Leaves
Tonka	*Dipteryx odorata*	Beans
Vanilla grass	*Anthoxanthum odoratum*	Grass blades
Vetiver	*Vetiveria zizanioides*	Root, essential oil
Wild gingerroot, Canada snakeroot	*Asarum canadense*	Root
Yellow sandalwood	*Santalum album*	Wood, essential oil

CHARACTERISTICS AND USES

SAFETY TIPS

CHARACTERISTICS AND USES	SAFETY TIPS
Sweet violet scent; excellent with other floral fragrances	Wear gloves when handling root, as it often causes skin irritation; use only in potpourris and sachets.
Rich, earthy scent when fresh; essential oil is very sharp and pungent; mellows after about 15 years	Safe for housekeeping uses.
Spicy, aromatic, and a bit fruity; essential oil is stronger, very pungent	Safe for housekeeping uses.
Woody; drier, much less sweet balsamic scent than yellow sandalwood; striking color	Safe for housekeeping uses.
Pleasant, vanilla scent	Possibly a skin irritant.
Newmown-hay, vanilla-like scent increases upon fermentation and drying	Safe for housekeeping uses.
Develops a much stronger, sweeter aroma when dry	Safe for housekeeping uses.
Light, pleasant, newmown-hay fragrance, increases when dry	Safe for housekeeping uses.
Sweet, newmown-hay fragrance; repels pests; loses sweetness with age	Safe for housekeeping uses. Keep beans from small children.
Newmown-hay, vanilla-like fragrance; grows in a mound shape, and thus more controllable in the garden than is sweet grass	Safe for housekeeping uses.
Dominant, strong, earthy, woodsy fragrance; use sparingly and then evaluate	Safe for housekeeping uses.
Spicy, earthy aroma with a skunky undertone; similar to but sweeter than valerian	Don't use the essential oil, which is carcinogenic to rodents, and so potentially dangerous to humans.
One of my favorites; sweet, rich, warm, soothing, and uplifting; very complementary to many other fragrance types	Safe as chipped wood, powder, or essential oil.

HERBAL
Resources

MAIL-ORDER SUPPLIERS

BOTTLES, MINERALS, AND OTHER SUPPLIES

The Dasun Company
P.O. Box 668
Escondido, CA 92033
Phone: 800-433-8929
Zeolite

Frontier Natural Products Cooperative
P.O. Box 299
Norway, IA 52318
Phone: 800-669-3275
Fax: 800-717-4372
Web site: www.frontiercoop.
  com
Bulk non-irradiated herbs, essential oils, fixed oils, glycerin, lanolin, amber and clear glass bottles, strainers, incense charcoals, loofahs, scrub brushes, natural soaps, and many other supplies

Internet, Incorporated
7300 49th Avenue North
Minneapolis, MN 55428
Phone: 800-328-8456
Fax: 612-971-0872
e-mail:
  www.netting@internet.com
FDA-approved plastic netting suitable for drying racks

Lavender Lane
7337 #1 Roseville Road
Sacramento, CA 95842
Phone: 888-593-4400
Fax: 916-339-0842
e-mail:
donna@lavenderlane.com
Web site:
www.lavenderlane.com
Bottles, essential oils, diffusers, fixatives, fixed oils, fullers earth, bentonite clay, lanolin, cocoa butter, beeswax, books; catalog: $2, refundable with order

Mid-Continent Agrimarketing, Inc.
1465 N. Winchester
Olathe, KS 66061-5881
Phone: 800-547-1392
Fax: 913-768-8968
Beeswax, paraffin, candle and soap molds, fixed oils, glycerin, glass bottles, metal and plastic bottle caps

SKS Bottle & Packaging, Inc.
3 Knavner Road
Mechanicville, NY 12118
Phone: 518-899-7488
Fax: 800-810-0440
e-mail: sales@sks-bottle.com
Web site: www.sks-bottle.com
Small, clear, amber, green, and blue glass bottles

HERB SEEDS AND PLANTS

Companion Plants
7247 N. Coolville Ridge Rd.
Athens, OH 45701
Phone: 740-592-4643
Fax: 740-593-3092
e-mail: complant@frognet.net
Web site: www.frognet.net/
  companion_plants

The Cook's Garden
P.O. Box 535
Londonderry, VT 05148-0535
Phone: 802-824-3400
Fax: 800-457-9705
e-mail:
www@cooksgarden.com
Web site:
www.cooksgarden.com

Goodwin Creek Gardens
P.O. Box 83
Williams, OR 97544
Phone: 541-846-7357
Fax: 541-846-7357

The Gourmet Gardener
8650 College Blvd., Suite 205
Overland Park, KS 66210
Phone: 913-345-0490
Fax: 913-451-2443
e-mail: information@
  gourmet-gardener.com
Web site: www.gourmet
  gardener.com

Harris Seeds
60 Saginaw Drive
P.O. Box 22960
Rochester, NY 14692-2960
Phone: 716-442-0410
Fax: 716-442-9386

J. L. Hudson Seedsman
Catalog requests (only):
P.O. Box 1058
Redwood City, CA 94064-1058
Catalog cost is $1.00
Other correspondence:
Star Rte. 2, Box 337
La Honda, CA 94020

Johnny's Selected Seeds
R.R. 1, Box 2580
Foss Hill Road
Albion, ME 04910-9731
Phone: 207-437-9294
Fax: 207-437-2165
e-mail:
staff@johnnyseeds.com
Web site:
www.johnnyseeds.com

Nichols Garden Nursery
1190 N. Pacific Highway
Albany, OR 97321-4580
Phone: 541-928-9280
Fax: 541-967-8406
e-mail:
info@gardennursery.com
Web site:
www.gardennursery.com

Park Seed
1 Parkton Avenue
Greenwood, SC 29647-0001
Phone: 800-845-3366
Fax: 800-209-0360
e-mail: info@parkseed.com
Web site: www.parkseed.com

Prairie Moon Nursery
R.R. 3, Box 163
Winona, MN 55987
Phone: 507-452-1362
Fax: 507-454-5238
e-mail: pmnrsy@luminet.net
Prairie plants, including sweet grass plugs

Richters Herbs
357 Highway 47
Goodwood, Ontario, L0C 1A0, Canada
Phone: 905-640-6677
Fax: 905-640-6641
e-mail: inquiry@richters.com
Web site: www.richters.com

The Sandy Mush Herb Nursery
316 Surrett Cove Road
Leicester, NC 28748-5517
Phone: 828-683-2014

The Seed Guild
P.O. Box 8951
Lanark ML11 9JG
United Kingdom
Web site: www.gardenweb.
  com/seedgd/list.html
Buys seed from botanic gardens all over the world and makes them available to both amateur gardeners and commercial outlets. Specializes in rare and unusual seeds. See web site for an online catalog.

Seeds of Change
P.O. Box 15700
Sante Fe, NM 87506-5700
Phone: 800-762-7333;
505-640-6677
Fax: 888-329-4762
e-mail:
gardener@seedsof-change.com
Web site:
www.seedsofchange.com

Shepherd's Garden Seeds
30 Irene Street
Torrington, CN 06790
Phone: 860-482-3638
Fax: 860-482-0532
e-mail:
garden@shepherd-seeds.com
Web site:
www.shepherd-seeds.com/

Territorial Seed Company
P.O. Box 157
Cottage Grove, OR 97424
Phone: 541-942-9547
Fax: 888-657-3131
e-mail: TSC@ordata.com
Web site:
www.territorial-seed.com

Underwood Gardens
4N381 Maple Avenue
Bensenville, IL 60106
Web site:
www.grandmas-garden.com

Well-Sweep Herb Farm
205 Mt. Bethel Road
Port Murray, NJ 07865
Phone: 908-852-5390
Fax: 908-852-1649

Herbal Periodicals

The Herb Companion, Interweave Press, 201 East Fourth Street, Dept. 0-B, Loveland, CO 80537-5655. Phone: 800-456-6018. Fax: 970-667-8317. Web site: www.interweave. com/iwpsite/herbie/herbie/http

The Herb Quarterly, P.O. Box 689, San Anselmo, CA 94960. Phone: 415-455-9540 Fax: 415-455-9541. e-mail: HerbQuart@aol.com. Web site: www.herbquarterly.com

Herbs for Health, Interweave Press, 201 East Fourth Street, Dept. 0-B, Loveland, CO 80537-5655. Phone: 800-456-6018. Fax: 970-667-8317. Web site: www.interweave. com/iwpsite/herbie/herbie/http

Books on Herbs

Berthold-Bond, Annie. *Clean & Green: The Complete Guide to Nontoxic and Environmentally Safe Housekeeping*. Woodstock, NY: Ceres Press, 1994. A useful guidebook.

Foster, Gertrude B., and Rosemary F. Louden. *Park's Success with Herbs*. Greenwood, SC: Geo. W. Park Seed Co., 1980. The first place I go to when I need reliable information about growing herbs.

Gruenberg, Louise M. *Potpourri, the Art of Fragrance Crafting*. Norway, IA: Frontier Cooperative Herbs, 1984. Learn to make potpourris that suit your sense of smell by coming up with your own variations of the base formulas.

Keville, Kathy, and Mindy Green. *Aromatherapy: A Complete Guide to the Healing Art*. Freedom, CA: Crossing Press, 1995. A fusion of herbalism and aromatherapy, with formulas for body care, medicinal herbs, perfumes, and even food recipes featuring essential oils.

Kowalchik, Claire, and William H. Hylton, eds. *Rodale's Illustrated Encyclopedia of Herbs*. Emmaus, PA: Rodale Press, 1987. A broad but thorough coverage of herbs.

Shaudys, Phyllis V. *Herbal Treasures*. Pownal, VT: Storey Books, 1990. Ideas and suggestions for herbal projects.

Steinman, David, and Daniel Epstein. *The Safe Shopper's Bible*. New York: Macmillan, 1995. A guide to what's safe and what's dangerous in the marketplace of cleaning and other products.

Acknowledgments

With thanks to my mother, Luise Ella Casazza Gruenberg, a woman who has always been willing to work twice as hard as anyone else to achieve perfection in her housework and who, when I wasn't interested in doing the same, recommended that I marry a rich man.

Thanks also to a man rich in everything that really matters, my husband, David James Walwark; and our children, Louisa Marie, Dave, Jr., and James Douglas Walwark, who, in keeping me busy cleaning up after them for years, inspired many of these solutions. Some day I'm going to move in with them, and let them clean up after me. Many thanks are also due to my gardening friends, Caron Raiche Wenzel and Charlene Jean Hanlon, who are always willing to share seeds, plants, books, knowledge, and their precious time with me.

Index

Page references in *italics* indicate illustrations;
page references in **bold** indicate tables.

Benzoin, **142–43**
Bible leaf. *See* Costmary
Bitter buttons. *See* Tansy
Black pepper, 14, 128
Blue gum eucalyptus *(Eucalyptus globulus)*, **61**
Borax, **136–37**
Boric acid, **136–37**
Boswellia carterii. See Frankincense
Bouncing bet. *See* Soapwort
Bran, **136–37**
Brandy mint. *See* Peppermint

C

Calamus *(Acorus* species), *34,* 34–35, **142–43**
  growing tips, 80, 83, 85
  in recipes, 98, 102, 121, 125, 131, 132
Calendula *(Calendula officinalis)*, 65, 106, 123
Camphor, white, 128, 129, **140**
Camphor basil *(Ocimum kilimand-scharicum)*, 32, *32*
Canada snakeroot. *See* Wild ginger
Candida, 36
Carnauba wax, **136–37**
Carpenter's weed. *See* Yarrow
Carpet cleaners, recipes, 100–103
Cashmere, cleaning tips, 111
Castile soaps, 95–96, **136–37**
Cat litter, clay-based, 136–37
Cedar, red. *See* Red cedar
Cerium Oxide Polishing Powder, 98
Chalk, **136–37**
Chamomile *(Matricaria recutita)*, 29, *35,* 35–36
  growing tips, 65, *75,* 78, *79*
  in recipes, 14, 18, 106, 123, 124, 125
Chenopodium ambrosiodes. See Epazoté
Cherry pie heliotrope, *75*
Christmas tree herb. *See* Sweet Annie
Chrysanthemum balsamita. See Costmary
Cinnamon leaf, **140**
Citric acid, 93, **136–37**
Citronella, **140**
Citrus fruit, 104, 124, 128, 131
Citrus solvent, **136–37**
Clary sage *(Salvia sclarea)*, 121, 123, **142–43**

Clove, 93, 128, 129, **140**
Cockroaches, herbs for, 33, 59, 103
Cocoa butter, **136–37**
Comfrey *(Symphytum officinale)*, 65, 107, 111
Commiphora myrrha. See Myrrh
Coneflowers *(Echinacea* species), 17, 65
Containers
  growing herbs in, 67, 73, *73*
  for storage, 19
Cooperative Extension Service, 29, 74
Copaiba balsam, **142–43**
Copal, 125, **142–43**
Costmary *(Chrysanthemum balsamita), 36,* 36–37
  growing tips, *79,81*
  in recipes, 103, 124, 131
Crafts, 34, 47, 52. *See also* Everlastings; Floral arrangements; Garlands; Ornaments; Tussie-mussies; Wreaths
Cream of tartar, **136–37**
Culpeper, Nicholas, 37

D

Damping-off prevention, 69
Daucus carota. See Queen Anne's lace
Decoction-infusion, 21, 124
Decoctions, 20–21, *21,* 84
Deer's tongue *(Trilisa odoratissima),* 132, **142–43**
Delicate fabrics, washing, 49, 115
Denatured alcohol, 12
Diatomaceous earth, **136–37**
Direct-seeding, *64,* 64–65
Disinfectant herbs, 14, 32, 52, 56, 59
Down, cleaning tips, 111
Dried herbs, formulating with, 17
Drying herbs, 84–87, *85,86*

E

E. coli, 52
Elder *(Sambucus nigra),* **61**
Elecampane *(Inula helenium), 37,* 37–38
  growing tips, 65, *81,* 83, 85
  in recipes, 132
Elf dock. *See* Elecampane

Tonka, **144–45**
Transplanting seedlings, 69–71, *70, 71*
Trees with herbal uses, 60, **61**
Trilisa odoratissima. See Deer's tongue
Tulsi. *See* Sacred basil
Turpentine, **138–39**
Tussie-mussies, 41, 45, 46, 50, 52

V
Vanilla grass, **144–45.** *See also* Sweet
grass
Velvet dock. *See* Elecampane
Vermiculite, **138–39**
Vetiver, 123, 128, **144–45**
Vinegar, 5, 15, 19, 24, 124
Vinegar extractions, 22
Viola tricolor. See Johnny-jump-up

W
Waldmeister (master of the woods). *See*
Sweet woodruff
Washing soda, **138–39**
Washing waters, sweet, 28, 29, 33
Water for formulas, 15
Watering plants, 72
Weeding plants, 72
White thyme, 14, 126
Wichtl, Max, 88
Wild bergamot. *See* Bee balm
Wild gingerroot, **144–45**

Wild sunflower. *See* Elecampane
Winter preparation, 72, *72*
Winter savory *(Satureja montana)*, 57,
57, 65, 77, 97
Witch hazel *(Hamamelis virginiana)*,
61
Woodrove. *See* Sweet woodruff
Woodwork cleaners, 103–9
Wools, cleaning tips, 111, 115
Wormseed. *See* Epazoté
Wormwood *(Artemisia absinthium)*, 28,
58, 58–59
growing tips, 65, *81*
in recipes, 18, 97, 98, 128
Woundwart. *See* Yarrow
Wreaths, 29, 31, 37, 39, 41, 42, 44, 45,
46, 48, 50, 52, 55, 56, 57, 58

Y
Yarrow *(Achillea millefolium)*, 28, 59,
59
growing tips, 65, 80, *81*
in recipes, 97, 98, 128
Yarroway. *See* Yarrow
Yellow sandalwood, **144–45**
Yucca *(Yucca glauca)*, 60, *60,* 83, 85,
109

Z
Zeolite, **138–39**